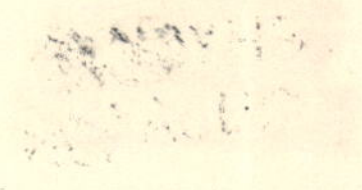

EXECUTIVES' HEALTH SECRETS

EXECUTIVES' HEALTH SECRETS

How to Lick Tensions and Pressures

BY

WILLIAM P. SHEPARD, M. D.

Former Medical Director of the Metropolitan Life Insurance Company

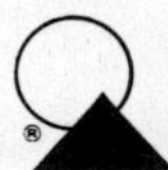

THE **BOBBS-MERRILL** COMPANY, INC.
A SUBSIDIARY OF **HOWARD W. SAMS & CO., INC.**
Publishers • INDIANAPOLIS • NEW YORK

First Printing

LIBRARY OF CONGRESS CATALOG CARD NUMBER 61-15538

DEDICATED TO

Frederic Hudson Ecker

HONORARY CHAIRMAN OF THE BOARD OF DIRECTORS
IN HIS EIGHTIETH YEAR OF ACTIVE
FULL-TIME SERVICE WITH THE
METROPOLITAN LIFE INSURANCE COMPANY

WITH THANKS

to

HARRIET

For encouragement, constructive suggestions and angelic patience with the 6:00 A.M. alarm clock, irregular meal times and the temperament of a writer-husband.

CONTENTS

FOREWORD

It has fallen to my lot, and a happy lot it's been, to work with and for business executives these many years. My observations are based not alone on my employer's executive family, who as a whole are a pretty healthy group, but on countless consultations with firms, large and small, over the country, with Chambers of Commerce, trade associations and committees of business executives who for one reason or another sought medical advice for the betterment of their own health, or that of their employees, or both. Since the advent of health insurance, both group and personal, I have watched the steady flow of claims filed in Home and Head Offices of the Metropolitan Life Insurance Company. Their analysis sheds much light on the extent and degree of various types of disability in different parts of the country from day to day and year to year.

I have come to regard the new medical specialty of industrial or occupational health as potentially one of the most promising fields for disseminating and demonstrating the great values of preventive medicine or, as I prefer to call it, health conservation. These values will never be fully realized, however, until (1) our physicians are better trained to recognize the existence of good health in its varying degrees and how to help the "healthy" individual conserve and enhance it; and (2) until more of the employers of the country have a better understanding of health conservation for their employees and themselves.

I have spent several years doing volunteer work along these lines for the medical profession and expect to continue. A logical place to start with employers, and through them all of industry, seems to be with the health of the executive himself. As a group, executives are showing an increasing concern with their own health which is all to the good. But they are assailed on every side with advice, some good, some bad. It is in the hope of dispelling some of their unnecessary fears and offering some common-sense suggestions based on sound medical tenets and long observation that this little book is written. It does not guarantee a long and healthy life. May it help you attain a happier one!

"My sword is Strength, my spear is Song;
With these upon a stubborn field
I challenge Falsehood, Fear and Wrong;
But Laughter is my shield."

ARTHUR GUITERMAN, "Re-armed"

EXECUTIVES' HEALTH SECRETS

A PRELIMINARY GLANCE

THE FIRST DUTY OF AN EXECUTIVE

Sometimes it seems as if the entire operation is the executive's duty. When something goes wrong he, or she, must know how to correct it, see that it is corrected, and then correct the cause of the error to avoid a recurrence. When something goes right, then it is time to plan ahead, develop new procedures and products, and the executive must direct the program. Personnel, finance, sales, plant, methods—all of these are the duty of the executive.

As a rule the executive has a family. It might well be said that there is where his duty lies.

To be selfish is one luxury the executive must deny himself. But it is not selfish to claim that his first duty is to himself.

To put a finer point on it, his first duty is to his good health. He must keep himself in perfect shape—or as close to perfect as possible. Perhaps perfection is always just one step beyond. No executive can allow himself to think he has achieved perfection. But with his health he must be close to it.

He must be not merely "okay," not "better thanks," not "getting along." He must be robust, alert, vigorous, cheerful and optimistic.

Look twice at the decision of the executive with an ulcer. It may be not the executive, but the ulcer, that makes the decision.

Rely not on the executive who suffers from chronic fatigue. He will postpone until tomorrow because today all he can think of is the rest he needs.

Blame not the executive with a splitting headache when she loses her temper; she is angry with it, not you.

Expect no dividends from the executive who fails to provide healthful working conditions, and an adequate industrial health program, for his employees. Either absenteeism or liability claims will make heavy inroads on his profits.

The first duty of an executive is to his own health, to assure that his mind will be clear, his nerves steady, and his stamina equal to the demands which will surely be put upon it.

And his next duty is to safeguarding the good health of his associates so that they may be equally able to perform their duties responsibly and thus place no unnecessary burdens on the executive.

WHO IS THE EXECUTIVE?

She may be the housewife tactfully and unobtrusively supervising children, husband, widowed mother and certain members of the garden club.

Or he may be the executive secretary of the local Junior Chamber of Commerce.

The drill-press operator is probably not an executive while on the job at his drill press, but at union headquarters, as chairman of a committee, he may well be.

In the main, however, by executive we mean just what you would expect—the head of a competitive enterprise in business or government. He is the president of the company, or a vice president or department head. He is an employer, with a payroll inexorably making its demands, competition ever lurking and menacing, and unpredictable markets. The executive is probably a man and that fact underlies much of the information in the pages that follow. But that women are taking an increasingly important role in business needs no supporting argument here, and the fact is recognized by giving her, the woman executive, a chapter of her own.

An executive is usually responsible for the performance of several or many other people, and therein lies his greatest problem. We can count on ourselves to do what we expect of us and if we fail we can justify the failure, but the unpredictability of what others may do puts a permanent strain on the adrenal glands, the nervous system, the whole pattern of our lives. The executive must see that those who report to him are functioning as they should, and this implies concern for their welfare as much as for the work done.

The executive also has someone to report to. It may be a superior in the company hierarchy or it may be the stockholders, or the customers. Whoever it is, it is often a heartless tyrant and a just cause for sleeplessness and anxiety.

Characteristically, the burdens of the executive are more than any one person can handle. He must learn to discriminate and to delegate; even then his troubles are intricate and numerous. These responsibilities impose a strain on his health and, where there is nothing more serious the matter, the executive is quite likely either to suffer from, or to be a candidate for, executivitis. This is bad enough in itself, and it can lead to worse.

It is hard to be an executive and not suffer from executivitis; therefore, the executive may have to learn to live with this chronic and characteristic state of health. If he does so, and it is the hope of this book to make it possible, the worst may be avoided.

DON'T COUNT YOURSELF OUT

Symptoms, causes and treatment of executivitis will be given further attention later on; briefly, now, drive, tension, indispensability—these are signs that the executive is an incipient patient. None of his business associates can help him in this condition. With the best of intentions they can only make it worse. The sooner he takes his doctor into partnership, the better for both of them. The doctor prefers prevention to cure—it is easier, safer and more practical—and prevention minimizes the suffering of the patient.

Let this be made clear now: there is no occupational hazard for the executive. It is not necessary that he suffer executivitis. A nervous breakdown is not an essential part of his career. The executive, who controls so many other significant activities, is not obliged to lose control of his own life or health. Statistics, and headlines, may indicate that executives suffer more and die younger than other mortals, but these statistics and headlines must be examined carefully. Executives are more prominent than porters and messengers and watchmen and file clerks. The executive's illness is reported; his employee's is not. Therefore, be not unduly alarmed if you happen to read about the hazards befalling numerous executive friends.

But though there is nothing to fear, there is much to watch out for. Drive, tension, indispensability—if you discover these signs in yourself, give your doctor a chance. Don't make it hard for him. Call him in early. And listen to what he has to say. It might be important to you.

THE MODERN DOCTOR

In my own lifetime I have seen a great change in the practice of medicine. The materials, techniques, facilities and assistants available to the modern doctor make it possible for him to claim with some justice that he is a scientist. Most doctors will still prefer to admit that they are subject to human fallibility. Nevertheless there is so much more available to them now than was at the command of a doctor at the beginning of the 20th century that the effectiveness of the doctor has more than doubled in that time.

And of all these improvements, the most important of all is the doctor's own attitude to his profession. Fifty years ago a doctor was proud if he could help hold an epidemic in check. Now his purpose is to prevent the start of a single illness, much less an epidemic.

Before soldiers go overseas they are given shots to protect them against germs they are likely to encounter. Diets are planned to be suitable for season and climate. The ounce of prevention worth the pound of cure is assiduously practiced. These procedures apply equally in industry. And the best way to apply them is to give the doctor—or the medical staff, if that is the fortunate situation—a sporting chance.

The modern doctor often works as one of a group in a clinic. He frequently seeks advice from specialists in other fields, or refers his patient directly to a specialist when that seems desirable. He has a well-equipped hospital at his service whenever he needs it. The drugs, vaccines and treatments available to him are truly miracle workers. All of this is a far cry from the call in the night, the dark and lonely country roads, and the emergency which had been allowed to develop so long that sometimes the assistance came too late and the doctor's effort was in vain, which was representative of the medical career in my father's time.

Later in this book I shall have more to say about how to choose a doctor. On the whole, I think you will find me quite broad-minded on the subject. It is of prime importance that the patient be satisfied with his choice and have confidence in his doctor and the advice he is receiving. The decision I leave to you; but I hope to give you a few helpful rules for making the right one. And I shall be satisfied if I make one lasting impression on you, which is that you should make your choice before the emergency, and thereafter consult your doctor regularly and freely.

The expense of medical attention should never be a matter of concern, whether it is for the company clinic or for the executive himself. It is easy enough to demonstrate that the cost of preventive medicine is actually one of the most sensible economies anyone can practice. As it applies to the executive himself, the question is less one of loss of productiveness; it is rather a matter of comparative efficiency. If he is to keep up with his competitors, the executive must operate at his peak form at all times. His doctor will help him to do this.

HOW MUCH OF HEALTH IS IN THE MIND?

Is it neurotic to be so concerned about health as to consult a doctor when we are feeling perfectly well? Or, by anticipating an ailment, by thinking about it too much, can we actually bring it on?

Hypochondria is frequently detected in their patients by doctors, of course, and executives, with their complex motivations, are peculiarly susceptible. Two points are important in this connection:

1. Let the doctor decide. If he tells you that your fears are unnecessary, that there is nothing more seriously wrong with you than being alive, and subject to the aches and pains of living, be-

lieve him and go your way rejoicing. But don't try to make the decision yourself. If you feel that something is wrong, there may be a reason for it. By questioning your doctor you may give him the greatest possible assist in the practice of his profession, which is early detection.

2. Never make the mistake of believing that mental, or mentally induced, or psychosomatic, illness is the same thing as imaginary illness. Mental illness is a very real thing and requires expert attention. Other illness may have psychosomatic causes; the headache, even the bad cold with sneezes and runny nose, may be caused by reluctance to face the conference scheduled for the morning. They are none the less real, the headache or the cold. Even more serious symptoms may develop if psychosomatic causes are consistently neglected.

Your doctor, because of the objectivity he can bring to the study of your case, and because of the comparisons he can make with similar cases in his practice, will help you to identify psychosomatic illness and its cause. Thereafter, you can learn to live with it.

No doctor can prevent the serious and difficult problems which are always being presented to the executive for solution. Fatigue, anxiety, stress will continue to take their toll. The executive understands that this is the life he has chosen, for the rewards it offers him. His resort to the doctor is not to eliminate his worries, but to assure that they do not compound to the point where they are no longer merely business problems, but become medical in nature.

Later we shall have more to say about how mental attitude can influence not only health but even success in business. The human mind, with its unfathomed resources of the unconscious, can be tricky. It's a good thing to know this, but it's nothing to worry about. Mind and body are one, and good health is a unity. With a sound mind and a strong body the executive's only fear is a falling away from this happy situation.

A nervous breakdown, the real thing, is something else again. This is difficult to anticipate, and even more difficult to handle when it occurs. The executive who feels that this possibility might become a reality in his life probably should give careful consideration to another means of livelihood. Certainly he should take the problem to his doctor, and give the doctor all the help he can in terms of frankness, in order to get from his doctor all the help he needs.

HOW THE BODY RESPONDS

One of the most interesting developments in modern medicine is the study of the relationship between physiology and environment. At times we hear some such statement as "If man will only live a natural life he will have no health problems."

Sounds plausible, on the face of it. Seems reasonable, that man is intended to be healthy (how else?) and when he is not, it is because of violation of some of nature's laws.

Here's the catch: a natural life as the phrase is used in this context must mean actually in a state of wild nature, the way lions and foxes and eagles live. Compared with the time it has taken for the development of his instincts, emotions and body reflexes, man's resort to shelter, clothing and an ordered way of life is but a fraction. Man suffers fears, anxieties and frustrations like his fellow animals, and he has, essentially, the same mechanisms for coping with these problems. But his responses must be different. He must exercise self-control.

He cannot live in a state of nature. As Robert Burns observed in *To a Mouse*:

> Still thou are blest, compar'd wi' *me*!
> The present only toucheth thee:
> But, Och! I backward cast my e'e,
> On prospects drear!
> An' forward, tho' I canna *see*,
> I *guess* an' *fear*!

The body's response to fear is a call for adrenalin in the blood to provide that extra power needed for the emergency. In frustration the body tenses the muscles to apply force to overcoming the obstacle. Emotions require great quantities of energy, which must be replaced either by rest or nutrition.

In a state of nature, Nature takes care of the body. The creature responds to the immediate situation without any complicating factors. Man must fight not only the situation, but himself as well. In fear he calls for calm courage, determination, or perhaps resignation. In frustration he calls for patience and imagination. To his emotions he applies perspective, and moderation.

Man cannot live in a state of nature, but he can learn to live in harmony with his physiology. Fear, frustration, high emotion, any kind of stress may serve a useful function. It is the abuse of the body which brings trouble. Worry, especially if prolonged, can do more harm than any crisis which is over and done with no matter what the result.

This as a good place to refer again to the woman executive. Does she worry more than her male counterpart? It would be quite an unsafe generalization to say so. The influence may be drawn that women tend to worry more than men because they often have less power to do something about a situation than the man has. The wife at home must rely on her husband to take the right course of action, and this may be good cause for worry. But the same does not apply to the woman executive.

She has the authority to act, and her judgment is often every bit as good as a man's. In some respects—in patience, sympathy, insight, in health and even in physical endurance—she may be better adapted to the demands of modern business than a man is. In Chapter 9 I show that the modern woman's health, stamina and longevity are superior not only to her men contemporaries, but to grandmother's, too.

From the point of view of health, there is little to choose between the male and female executive. Other factors of temperament, experience and motivation may affect the qualifications for certain positions, but these are not the concern of the doctor, unless perhaps, occasionally, the psychiatrist.

Except where sexual differences obviously apply, as in time out for maternity, considerations of health apply equally to the male or female executive. And, again, except where sexual differences obviously apply, as prostatitis, the pages which follow are intended for both men and women even though they seem directed to men because men are still in the majority in business.

OVERWEIGHT

Women as a rule take better care of themselves than men do, and the woman executive who is seriously overweight is comparatively rare. The women who characteristically weigh too much have idleness to blame. Indisposed to exercise because they are out of the habit, or were never in it, and without other interests to distract them, they become self-indulgent.

Overweight is a health hazard, and makes a poor insurance risk, in any circumstances. A lean horse for a long race is still a good maxim. Boys need more food than girls, but when he becomes a man and follows a sedentary life, the executive should remind himself that this need no longer holds. The woman executive is usually conscious, and therefore considerate, of her figure. The man is likely to be more careless, though he should not be. Not only is he less attractive to women with a paunch and three chins, he is less efficient, less enduring, and the strain on his heart is almost certain to influence his life span.

Sometimes the fat executive eats too much as a compensation for self-denial of other pleasures. Eating and drinking are undeniably very real pleasure of life, and in Chapter 5 I have some comments on drinking which I hope will be encouraging for those who enjoy it. Do read this section carefully, I beg of you, and bear in mind that my plea is always for moderation.

There is encouragement for the fat man, too, because there are ways of losing weight without denying oneself all the pleasures of the table. In fact, the crash diet is seldom desirable, and should never be taken except under the direct supervision of a physician. With adequate vitamins, and a properly balanced diet, eating should remain a pleasure without becoming a source of worry. In this respect, his doctor can be of immediate help to his executive patient who is otherwise in perfect health.

KEEPING THE INSTRUMENT TUNED

Part and parcel with diet in its effect on weight goes exercise. I have heard it argued that exercise can have little influence on the executive's body weight, and it is true that a lot of hard physical work is required to undo the damage wrought by just a few extra calories at meal time. For the executive, who must expect to spend much of his time in a restraining environment, exercise alone cannot be relied on to keep the weight in line.

It should also be remembered that exercise, by using up energy, has a tendency to stimulate the appetite. After a good workout it is easy to feel so good that enthusiasm for eating overcomes all built-in restraints, and the end result of exercise is increased weight.

The executive must also remind himself that he is no longer an athlete. Even the junior executive must realize that he quickly loses that condition he gained at the training table, and that strained and complaining muscles are the least he can expect in damage from overdoing it. The athletics of youth are not for the executive, not even if he is a football coach. But some form of *regular* exercise is important for the maintenance of good health, as I describe in Chapter 6.

This is important not only in keeping the weight down, but also in aiding all the other natural functions of the body and its organs. The bowels, the kidneys, the liver, the lungs, even—mark this—the mind, all operate better with the benefit of some physical exersize. Exhaustion, even fatigue, means that the exercise is excessive. It should be just enough to produce a stimulation, a feeling of pleasure in being alive.

Nourishment, exercise and rest, not too much of any, but all in proper balance, these are the ingredients which make the successful and happy executive.

AN INDUSTRIAL HEALTH PROGRAM

The good health of the executive himself is one of the first requirements for the health and happiness of the workers in his charge. If his health is adequate to give him the strength he needs to meet all the demands on him for patience, endurance and energy, then he will not be an "ulcer-maker" among his employees. And one of the best provisions he can make to assure that he will be this kind of executive is an adequate industrial health program.

This will depend, of course, on the size and kind of the operation, and its location. In some industries there are built-in hazards to health; the most notorious of these, atomic energy, requires all kinds of safeguards. But even in white-collar offices where danger of any kind is at a minimum there will be advantages in a planned program.

This may require a full-time staff or, at the other extreme, a part-time nurse may be sufficient. Not only does an industrial health program reduce the chances of accident, and cut down loss of time on account of illness, but it contributes to the efficiency and happiness of the executive through the peace of mind it brings him.

In this book you will notice that I continuously advocate reference to your doctor for advice before the need for his services becomes desperate. I am sure you will understand that there is no economic motivation about this. I am by no means trying to drum up trade for the doctor who is probably already overworked anyway. What I am trying to do is to put the teamwork between doctor and patient on the highest possible level, so that each will help the other at his best.

Nowhere do I consider this counsel from the physician more important than in the use of the many props our civilization offers to help get us through the day. In recent years many new drugs, tranquilizers and stimulants have been developed. Properly administered they are extremely useful, but more for the curing of serious ills than in getting through the cares of day. Follow strictly the instructions of your doctor in the use of sleeping pills, tranquilizers and stimulants.

We have long known, of course, that care should be observed in the use of the familiar stimulants and sedatives: coffee, tea, alcohol and tobacco. These can be friends of the executive when properly used. The results of their abuse, especially alcohol and tobacco, can be tragic.

INDISPENSABILITY

Drive, tension, indispensability are the symptoms of executivitis, especially indispensability. Sometimes this is real; the executive has reserved for himself all authority in the company and nothing can happen when he is away. In other cases the indispensability is more imaginary. Either way, it is just as serious from the medical point of view.

Although his position is important, his experience valuable, his decisions wise, and his authority real, it is a superior executive who plans for the day when he can put it all behind him by retirement. The sooner the better. To retire early is one of the better ways of avoiding that untimely death in harness that makes unpleasant headlines.

The executive need not fear the demoralizing results of idleness in retirement because it is not necessary to be idle. By-products of a successful career should be so many side interests that there will be time enough in the day, or the year, to attend to them all. That the business can prosper without him may be something of a shock, but of a kind that will be good for him. If he can survive that, he can survive anything.

CHAPTER 1

EXECUTIVITIS: ITS PREVENTION AND CURE

ONE of the most curious things about executives whom I have known, worked for, observed, admired, been amused and harassed by, advised and ministered to these many years, is—How do they get that way? Thank goodness they do get that way. If they hadn't we might have missed the amazing progress which has characterized this daring but still infantile experiment in democracy called the U.S.A. But what makes some men, and some women, get the urge to become superior to others, to seek added responsibility, to study harder and work harder than others, and to climb and climb until they get to the summit of their own particular ambition, and even then often seek other and higher summits?

WHAT IS EXECUTIVITIS?

Is it all greed for more money and more power? It can't always be, because many of them really do amazing things: build railroads, skyscrapers and bridges; manufacture necessities and luxuries cheaper and better; organize big businesses which benefit their customers and stockholders alike. Of course, there are the greedy and unscrupulous among them, but in my observation, especially in recent years, they are in the minority.

Could it be that the production of executives in this and the other free countries is one of the characteristics of western freedom? Is that one of the many things that differentiate us most markedly from the Marx-Lenin-Stalin philosophy of Communism?

In his revealing book *The Future is Ours, Comrade,* Joseph Novak quotes a former Soviet army officer who tells of being victimized by a counter-intelligence unit. After being sent to hard labor at the Manchurian frontier, he set about bettering his impaired record by very hard work and did so. But this bitter lesson taught him that "a kind heart does not pay. The most important thing in life is to perform your duties according to the rules set by society. I came," he says, "to understand that they were not made for some miserable individual like me to try to improve them on his own. Now I'll remember for the rest of my life that if you try to help someone, the most you can do is to harm yourself." Novak goes on to illustrate the fact that conformity with the rules laid down by one's superiors is the better part of discretion under Communism.

Under such rules, could this country have produced that curious but invaluable person, The Executive? No, we still have ample proof that the boy or girl with superior talents here can, by using those superior talents and barring misfortune, become a most productive and valuable citizen. To be sure, some fall by the wayside. Others succumb to the temptation of making a "quick buck" regardless of ethics. But what other country, without the hereditary advantage of an earldom or a military reward from the Crown, could have produced an Edison, an Alexander Bell, a Kettering, a Henry Ford, the Wright Brothers, a Rockefeller and many other great leaders who, by dint of hard work and a free enterprise system to work in, became Executives?

My thesis here is that The Executive, be he president of a large company, or a shop foreman responsible for an important unit of production, or a bank teller whose integrity and the integrity of those he supervises must be beyond question, are all precious to our society. They are worth producing, nurturing and preserving from executivitis.

Executivitis may be described briefly as that state of mind which stems from egocentricity (focus on self) to an abnormal degree. It produces feelings of omniscience, great power over subordinates, ability to solve all problems without study or consultation (often according to whim), know-all, see-all, the Devil take the hindmost, and the public be damned. We all know this type of executive. He's got it! Executivitis!

It's hard to cure at this stage, short of being carried out bodily. It could have been prevented but long, long ago. It's interesting, but tragic, to see this condition of executivitis from a doctor's standpoint when the "know-all, see-all" becomes ill. He's frightened beyond reason. He must be back in the office in the morning or he'll get another doctor! At that point I, having less patience than most of my respected colleagues, bow out and say, "Goodnight, Mr. Executivitis." He may then lay his soul bare. If you listen carefully, you find that he is scared. He always has been scared. He is really a very insecure person at heart. By bellowing his orders, displaying his dollars, having his own way no matter what, he has been able to bolster his ego and maintain his supremacy to the great comfort of his ego. This conduct reassures him. His image of himself is that he is a great man!

But now he has a pain, an awful pain. He thinks he may die. Dollars and bellicosity and throwing his usually excessive weight about will not relieve that pain. For the first time in many years, he pleads for someone to help him. To the observant doctor he is unfrocked—just another human being with the same vulnerabilities as the rest of us: upset stomach, growling intestines, thickened arteries, strained heart and swollen feet.

Ofttimes he can be cured of his immediate complaint: a touch of indigestion, a spasm or a kink somewhere in his overworked gastro-intestinal tract, a kidney stone perhaps (which really gives him a right to scream), or even a full-blown coronary. These and other common ailments of all humans can usually be relieved, often cured, and the individual in pain and apprehension can always be comforted. But the executivitis—that's another matter. Chances are when you get the kinks out of his intestine, or the stone out of his bladder, he will return to his old compulsive pattern of working and bolstering his voracious ego. He may possibly come out of it chastened, ready to look at himself squarely and change his way of life. It's worth trying in every case, despite the time, patience and almost psycho-analytical understanding it demands of the doctor. If friendly rapport can be established, if the executive is really scared enough, if he develops confidence and genuine liking for his doctor, that doctor may be the one and only person who can cure his executivitis. But it's awfully hard to change the habits of a lifetime. Chances are he will go right back to being THE Big Brass.

Executivitis is much easier to prevent than to cure.

PUBLIC IMAGE OF THE EXECUTIVE

This tycoon tends to represent the public image of The Executive today, especially by some of the leaders of the Democratic Party. He is to be distrusted as a despoiler of those who toil. He is thought to be a clever one at finding ways to elude the income tax. He wants to see the governmental budget balanced, an old fashioned idea if he would but heed the neo-economists and let the government do more for the people paying for it by increasing taxes still more. He is a mortal enemy of the Unions. He is ever ready to curry the favor of people high in governmental positions by arranging yacht trips, paying hotel bills and giving away Persian rugs. He is entrenched greed personified.

This is an unfortunate confusion in the minds of some of the public. They think they see in this pattern, The Executive. What they really see is a man with executivitis.

Well, even the most advanced cases of executivitis were seldom quite that bad, though a few were, and still are. But they tend to be the old fashioned kind. They were the tycoons of yesteryear who operated in quite a different milieu than that of today. They preceded, and a few survived the "trust-busting" of Theodore Roosevelt. And even he, it may be recalled, was living in a day when "might was right," when battleships were sent to rescue United States citizens who were abused by foreign powers, when "The Marines have landed and all is secure." Incidentally, one wonders how he and the public of his day would have reacted to the insults of a Khrushchev or a Castro. How much the world and especially the Western World attitudes have changed since then! And how much The Executive of western big business has changed too!

Not all of those older tycoons were so bad as some of the public pictured them. Not all had executivitis. They did seem to be the monarch of all they surveyed. They often gave orders which no one had the courage to question, lest he incur the tornado of "the old man's" wrath. They may have seemed tough on some of their subordinates, but some feel even today that the first responsibility of the employer is to teach his employees to do a decent day's work. They did get things done, however, to the great benefit of the public, their employees and, not incidentally, themselves.

There are still a few of this species around and I, for one, hope they may be preserved. They are powerful, colorful, interesting and often capable of enormous generosity. They pursue an interesting philosophy, namely, that they don't need the advice of committees to run their business—expert consultants, yes, but committees, no, since they nearly always come out with a compromise recommendation which satisfies neither party to a controversy. These executives illustrate the philosophy that any decision is often better than no decision, and that anyone whose decisions are 50 per cent correct is doing all right. They do not have executivitis—not very badly at least. They, like the modern executive, are really supermen, physically and mentally.

THE MODERN EXECUTIVE

The modern executive is quite a different person from his predecessors. He is likely to be younger, he is studious, hard working, soberly aware of his heavy responsibilities but not oppressed by them. He is more likely to consult his carefully picked subordinates, basing his decisions on a careful study of all the factors involved. But he realizes that when all the facts are assembled and verified, there may still be room for a difference of opinion between his advisors and that he and he alone must often make the final decision and take full responsibility for it. And I like to think that his decisions are more often right than wrong, based as they are on study, not whim or intuition.

The modern executive, including the heads of departments to whom fullest possible authority is delegated, works longer hours than his predecessor. This is in interesting contrast to his employees, who through union contracts or otherwise, are paid more for fewer hours and less output. He works longer hours despite the fact that the more money he makes, the greater are his taxes, so that he has much less take-home pay than his predecessor of fifty years ago. He is often a lonely man, since the number of his social and financial co-equals and companions diminishes the higher he climbs.

But he may worry more frequently about his health, partly because we all seem to think more about our health than formerly, partly because so much health advice is thrown at us, some good, some bad. Mostly, perhaps, he is more concerned about his health because so much is made of the early death or illness of his contemporaries. Much has been said and written about the stress and strain of being an executive, the inference being that it is overwork that causes the ulcer or the early heart attack.

THE EXECUTIVE HAS NO OCCUPATIONAL HAZARDS

And here cometh the first lesson: There is no discernible occupational hazard connected with the job of being an executive. Studies by the medical directors of large companies, as well as studies of occupational mortality (such as they are in this country) fail to show that the executive dies younger or suffers many more or many different impairments and disabilities than his fellow workers. Even stomach ulcers, once said to be an executive's disease, are no more common among executives than others; in fact, in some studies they are less so. Coronary disease and other heart attacks are by no means more common in the executive than anyone else, except women in general. Women have lower death rates than men, longer life span, and considerably less disease of the heart and blood vessels.

But to find that the executive is not "burning himself out" with stress and strain and overwork, and especially ulcers, is a blow to the type of tycoon still extant who is quoted as saying to his business partner "This fellow Jives looks like a very valuable man, but we can't possibly promote him yet, he hasn't even had one ulcer."

In fact there is some reason to believe that the successful executive of today (and this may have been true yesterday too) is in truth a superman, both physically and mentally. He is a doer, despite obstacles which seem insurmountable to others. He gets things done despite the frailties and stupidity of his subordinates. He manages by consultation, expert advice, uncanny resourcefulness and great drive to overcome the handicaps of mounting taxes, increasing labor costs, grueling competition, to bring his company out on top. He and his ilk are largely responsible for U.S. supremacy in commerce, industry, invention and output.

But here's the funny thing: He goes charging ahead trying to prove himself a superman when it is already apparent to all about him. The harder he works, the less he has to live on; the higher he goes, the fewer real friends he has, including his family.

Though he is obviously a superman, it is a strange paradox that he largely disregards the few simple rules of healthful living, and yet is often unduly concerned, bemused and confused about his own health. He is still susceptible to executivitis.

The preservation of good health, the attainment of even better health, and the quickest possible restoration of good health once it has been lost—all these have been cloaked in mystery since the age of the tribal witch doctor. There are still many mysteries which take place in that old bag called the human integument, which puzzle the wisest modern doctors. But there are likewise many discoveries which have taken away some of the mysteries. They have become just plain facts of life. A simple explanation of some of the "plain facts" which seem especially relevant to the health of the executive, may provide some immunity from executivitis to present and future executives, both male and female.

SCAREHEADS SELL PAPERS

Such headlines as "Young Executive Dies on Golf Course," "Rising Young Business Man Suffers Heart Attack," "Untimely Death of Famous Playwright," are unsettling, especially when the deceased is a friend or contemporary. In fact they may scare the "hell" out of you, and if the "hell" consists of total ignorance about, and neglect of your health, it may be a good thing.

During a convention of some 1,500 district managers from all parts of the country, one of the younger of them dropped dead. In the next three days the medical department of that company had over two hundred requests for physical examinations from the visitors. Most of them had been offered their annual examination paid for by their company during the preceding year, but had either declined or neglected it.

The irony of it is, the man who died had had his annual physical examination just before leaving his home, and, as they so often say, "he was pronounced perfectly healthy." This sort of thing happens often enough to justify some explanation. Here's why:

PERIODIC PHYSICAL EXAMINATION NOT A GUARANTEE OF IMMORTALITY

Important and helpful as it is, the periodic physical examination is not a guarantee of immortality, or, in fact, of any certain remaining span of life. Things do occasionally go wrong with the heart or brain or other vital organs which cannot be foreseen or predicted by the most skilled of physicians and the most extensive of laboratory tests. The periodic examination has other important values which we shall see later, but it is not a ticket to immortality.

MORTALITY TABLES ARE INEXORABLE

Those life insurance actuaries who are often accused of having stones for hearts (but who also die of heart failure even as other mortals) will say that, given 100,000 individuals at various ages, they can tell you with reasonable accuracy how many will die each year. And so they can! They can tell you how many, but not who. Death rates from specific causes of death as well as total death rates change from time to time—usually for the better in this country—but one thing is sure: the death rate among 100,000 individuals in 150 years will be 100 per cent—that is, until we discover some new elixir of everlasting life.

For men now age 35, the chances of surviving to age 96 are 7 in 1,000. So likewise, the chances of living to age 50 are 934 in 1,000. The grim reaper's scythe catches just so many each year of life, more at the very young ages, fewer in youth and early adulthood, and more and more each year after fifty. You can't change this over-all picture. But you and your doctor can often increase the odds in your favor by the application of a sensible regime of living.

My point here is that the death of prominent business men of any age is more likely to result in an obituary in the press than the death of an able-bodied seaman or a dock worker or a farm laborer of similar age. Thus we get the impression that young businessmen are dying off in droves, or that heart attacks are becoming much more common. The first impression is false, they are not dying off in droves. The second impression, that heart attacks are becoming more common, is correct. But that is because more people have escaped earlier death from diphtheria, tuberculosis or typhoid fever, and are living to the heart disease age.

As to those seemingly inexplicable deaths of relatively young friends, many of them are not so inexplicable if an autopsy is done. Some had rheumatic or scarlet fever in childhood, leaving them with a permanent defect in one or another of the heart valves. Some, we find, really lived to a remarkable age, considering the type of congenital heart or blood vessel defect they had. Others had an unhappy combination of genes in their parents or grandparents which made them more susceptible to arterial degeneration or cardiac collapse.

And here cometh the second lesson: To be a really successful and healthy executive, one should choose his parents and grandparents with great care.

IMPORTANCE OF HEREDITY

Hereditary tendencies, or weaknesses can often be overcome, or bolstered or adjusted to, so that they become almost no handicap at all. And we must be pretty sure what is really a hereditary handicap and what is not. Many undesirable personality traits which repeat themselves for several generations are not hereditary at all. They can be recognized early and overcome by early child training and enlightened self-discipline.

For example, suppose the father of the family has a quick temper, given to outbursts of anger at the children, his wife and his subordinates. His mother, if living, will say "John's just like his father was, quick to anger, quick to forgive." The wife takes up the refrain, defending and excusing Daddy before the children. The oldest daughter, we'll say, who tends to "take after" her father, decides this is a pretty good way to get attention, and even get away with murder, so to speak. Whereupon she begins to enjoy temper tantrums "just like her Daddy." Wise parents can stop this "hereditary curse" if the father will watch the example he sets for the children a little more carefully and both parents will agree to walk out of the room when little sister has a temper tantrum, finding some other way to give her the attention which she craves.

The point here is that the so-called quick temper is not hereditary. It is the product of the environment in which the child is reared. And that environment can be controlled much more easily than can the genes in the sperm and the ovum.

Among the handicaps that may, though not always, be hereditary, as a good example for the purpose of our discussion here, is deafness coming on in middle life and becoming progressive. This does not necessarily strike each generation, and by no means does it strike each individual. When it does occur, however, and the individual and his doctor are on the alert for it, there should be no delay in starting training with a suitable hearing aid. And training it takes, much more so than with a pair of glasses. Early attention and prompt action here will permit the modern executive to escape the condition that forced his grandfather's retirement because "he couldn't hear what they were saying about him."

Fortunately the individual with certain obvious hereditary limitations almost automatically chooses a vocation or profession which will minimize his handicap. To come back to progressive deafness, it was unfortunate for him, but fortunate for the rest of the world that Beethoven chose a musical career almost to the exclusion of everything else. He died at a fairly early age totally deaf, embittered and frustrated. A hearing device, had it been available then, together with a deliberate effort on his part to develop other absorbing interests might have prolonged his life and certainly would have given comfort to his declining years. What he lacked was modern medical equipment and advice.

The son of a college professor showed unmistakable signs of brilliance by the age of three years. But he was a rather sober, studious and curious child, with little interest in the games of exercise enjoyed by his young friends. Instead of berating him, and making his young life miserable by urging him to "get out and play with the boys," the professor consulted the family doctor whose careful examination showed the possibility of a congenital heart defect. More careful and thorough cardiac examination confirmed this diagnosis by the age of five. It was decided, however, that the defect was so slight that no surgery was indicated, since the small foramen in the wall between the ventricles would probably close itself as he grew older. Thus, the boy and his parents are satisfied to let him develop his remarkable mental abilities without trying to make him an athlete. Thus, too, he was saved the fate that overtook one of his cousins with a similar but unrecognized heart defect, who died at seventeen during a strenuous athletic contest.

So from the standpoint of heredity, with respect to your health and physical and mental endowments, what is done is done. We must make do with what we have. And what we have may not be so bad after all if we have some understanding of our limitations, how to live with them and make the best of them.

SOME SENSIBLE HEALTH GUIDES

Before suggesting some simple guides to health, let us first see what we mean by health. It is not merely absence from disease, which is good enough in itself, but also attaining a state of well-being both physically and mentally which will permit the individual to function to his maximum capacity within his inherent limitations, and which will permit as long and happy a life as possible.

Obviously, no set of rules will guarantee this sublime state to anyone, but in my opinion, based on observation and such medical knowledge as I may have, the following suggestions will be helpful.

1. *Have a good doctor.*

There never was a time in the world's medical history when a physician could be more valuable than now. The modern physician has more skill and knowledge than any of his predecessors. He also has more scientific aids in the hospital and laboratory than his forefathers.

We often long for the "old fashioned family doctor." Well, he and his little black bag are gone with his horse and buggy. Willing, ready and comforting as he was, he didn't know much compared with present day knowledge—and we didn't treat him very well. He often worked over seventy hours a week and he was lucky if he collected his reasonable fees for 50 per cent of the work he did. This is because many people in the days of the horse and buggy doctor considered calling the doctor a last resort. This was an expense they had hoped to avoid. There was no provision for it in their budget, if they had one. They would resort to home remedies, accept medical advice from the neighbors, seek diagnosis and treatment from the druggist and buy gallons of patent medicines before they called the doctor. They would call a veterinarian for their sick cattle much more readily than call a physician for Mary's persistent cough, which often turned out to be tuberculosis. Unfortunately there are still people today who feel the same way. They avoid the doctor like the plague.

These are not times to be niggardly on medical advice and care. The modern physician has too much to offer in the way of preventive and curative services to be relegated to the court of last resort. But, alas, too many people will readily pay for regular servicing and inspection of their automobile, while neglecting the servicing and inspection of their most valuable and totally irreplacable mechanism, the body.

The horse and buggy doctor's wonderful attributes of kindliness, understanding and dedication to his patients are still preserved in the best of modern physicians, and these attributes are supplemented by scientific diagnostic and curative aids totally lacking in that little black bag.

How to choose, use and not abuse your modern physician will be fully discussed in Chapter 2.

2. *Learn to prefer moderation to excesses*

This is the one rule for modern healthful living that I would put above all others next to having a good doctor. Its frequent violation usually stems from thoughtlessness, or ignorance which we shall try to dispel in Chapter 3. Its violation sometimes stems from rather deep psychological causes which we shall try to explain, and hopefully dispel, in Chapter 6.

3. *Understand yourself*

This is a little like saying "stop worrying," a futile dictate like "stop breathing." Nevertheless, it seems apparent to me that many executives and would-be executives could understand themselves better and to their great advantage if only they would set about it. Why do you want to be Number One man? Are you *sure* you know? Do you fully realize that you may not be a sow's ear, exactly, but you'll never be a silk purse? On the other hand, are you aware that you may have at hand all the materials to make a silk purse if only you use them and put them together right? Do you know that to become Number One man requires a great deal of continuous self-schooling and self-discipline? Have you now, or can you acquire, what it takes? We will discuss that in Chapter 4.

4. *Learn what makes you "tick"*

Besides a few basic principles of psychology, referred to above, the superman, which the good executive must be, should know something about what makes the body function as well as it does, so that he may discern the fallacy in false health claims, avoid the things that unnecessarily disturb this marvelous living machinery with which he is endowed, and understand with some intelligence the advices given by his doctor.

It is not hard to understand the fundamental principles of nutrition, metabolism, procreation and the like. Trouble is, many of us were conditioned against these things by poorly taught courses in high school or college, variously called "Hygiene," "Health Education," "Physical Education," etc. While this short book cannot be a text on physiology and psychology combined, some of the more important points will be covered in Chapter 6.

5. *Make the best of what you have*

This would seem almost a fundamental law of nature and of survival. Yet it is often more manifest in animals than in humans.

None of us is born perfect. We all have limitations of one kind or another. Some we can overcome; many we can't. It is important for each individual to recognize his limitations and make the best of them. Those that cannot be overcome may actually be turned to our advantage. Most people who are color blind do not know it until someone gives them a color test. They have not been aware of, or handicapped by, this condition. They have automatically made the best of what they have. Actually, they adjust so well that they can do almost anything but cable-splicing and rug-weaving. Many with serious physical impairments actually capitalize on them. Others withdraw to a life of frustration and self-pity. This is elaborated in Chapter 8.

6. *Learn to set yourself a realistic pace*

We doctors see so many people who were born to be good basset hounds but are trying to be greyhounds. Each individual has his own natural pace, within which he can remain healthy and get lots done. Most folks can speed up, or work long hours for temporary periods. But some, having done this, get the foolish notion that they are greyhounds and can continue this pace indefinitely. Hard work, *per se*, for temporary periods never killed anybody. It's not the pace that kills; it is a continuous excessive pace and one's attitude toward it. Relaxation, delegation of authority, vacations and avoidance of tensions are discussed in Chapter 7.

7. *Finally—Have fun!*

There's no sin in having wholesome fun, despite the teachings of some of our puritanical forefathers to the contrary. This, too, is further discussed in Chapter 7.

CHAPTER

2

HOW TO CHOOSE, USE, AND ABUSE YOUR DOCTOR

To START with, let me admit that I could be suspected of being a special pleader with a built-in bias on this subject. If that be true, my only defense is: who wouldn't be if they had seen what I have over the years? As the Negro spiritual goes, "Nobody knows the troubles I've seen—Nobody knows but Jesus."

THE CASE FOR CALLING A DOCTOR

One reason I gave up the private practice of medicine in the beautiful fertile, rolling hills of northwestern Iowa was the great number of people who came into my office, and my father's before me, who were doomed to die, despite our most heroic efforts, because they had not come to the doctor soon enough.

In those days a ruptured appendix carried a high mortality and we saw plenty of such cases because the victims called the doctor too late. We still lacked the toxoid to prevent diphtheria, but we could nearly always cure it with anti-toxin if we got the case early enough. To be called to the farmhouse after one child had been ill a week and the other children were just coming down with diphtheria meant sending the father by horseback or buggy, post-haste into town for a supply of anti-toxin while I settled down for the rest of the day and night with a machine to generate bromine gas which was then brought to "loosen the diphtheritic membrane" obstructing the child's windpipe. There was no hospital within thirty miles and the roads were often considered impassable by everyone but the doctor.

I would lay out my instruments ready to try to insert a tube through the larynx, or if that failed, to cut a hole in the windpipe in the hope of getting below the membrane for the life-giving air. I shall never forget my first success with the tracheotomy, hearing the air hungrily sucked into that tube in the neck and watching the poor little one's cheeks turn from blue-black to fresh pink again. I wish I could forget my failures, where the membrane literally filled the upper bronchial tubes while I stood helpless watching the child smother. There was one winter when we had, my father and I, twenty such deaths. I thought bitterly, "When will these ignorant fools ever learn to call the doctor in time."

"Chronic pregnancy," as we called it, was the chief reason for calling the doctor, although delivery by a doctor was still considered a luxury by many a farmer. Many relied solely on a "neighbor woman." Some tempered this spendthrift tendency by not calling the doctor until the last possible minute, knowing that if he didn't get there until the baby was born, he could not charge the usual $10 delivery fee. There was many a time when I arrived just as the head was presenting, hardly having time to wash my hands. These were the lucky cases and most of mine were that way. But to enter a stuffy farmhouse and find a woman I had never seen before already in labor and having convulsions from eclampsia was a problem I dreaded to face. Too often it resulted in loss of both the mother and baby. Deaths from eclampsia can usually be prevented if the mother is seen early enough and the doctor is prepared for this emergency.

Among the most tragic cases of that day were the young adults who died of tuberculosis. I considered myself well qualified to diagnose early tuberculosis, and there was a good state-operated sanatorium available. But I never saw an early case. All were far advanced by the time they decided to take their months-old cough to a doctor. Most of them had exhausted the extensive cough syrup armamentarium of the drug store while their tubercle bacilli merrily multiplied until a cure was seldom seen. Also, there was considerable resistance to going to the sanatorium. Nearly all the people they knew who went there stayed a few months and came home to die.

Smallpox, typhoid fever, pneumonia and cancer were always with us, leaving their dead behind and the overworked doctor handicapped by being called too late.

I decided, therefore, to specialize in public health and preventive medicine, applying them in succession to health departments, voluntary organizations devoted to the health education of the public and in more recent years, to industry. This was a great disappointment to my father, who, though he never said so, I think considered me the black sheep of a long line of physicians in private practice. He would say to me as we were walking down the street: "See that man over there? Last year, he fell into the threshing machine and I saved his life. In public health work you may save some lives, but how can you tell who?" Of course, I couldn't. But I know I have helped others in preventive medicine save many, many lives, even though those who were saved don't know that, but for our efforts, they might have been among my earlier patients who died of diphtheria, smallpox, typhoid fever and tuberculosis. It has been a satisfying life-work, and upon that rests this built-in bias regarding the value of having a good doctor and calling him early.

I know a doctor's services cost money, and sensible people have an aversion for spending money unnecessarily. But my contention is that the doctor is worth it, especially with the modern superbly trained physician, and especially for the modern invaluable business executive.

People also have an aversion for preparing for unpleasant eventualities. The thought of death is unpleasant; hence they fail to make wills or buy enough life insurance. The thought of illness is unpleasant; hence they give no thought to how the good doctor might help them avoid it, or at least minimize the degree of disability it causes.

In the world's history of medicine there never was such a time as the present. The modern doctor is better trained, has more knowledge and skill and more scientific methods of diagnosis and treatment than any of his predecessors. Now is the time for you to select your doctor if you have not already done so. How do you go about this? Do you want a general practitioner, obstetrician, pediatrician or other specialist? Have you recently moved into a new community, leaving the old medical affiliations behind? This chapter will give some sensible and practical suggestions on how to go about choosing your physician, and how to use him best, once he is chosen.

HOW DOCTORS ARE USUALLY CHOSEN

The American Medical Association says all doctors are good, providing they have passed their state board examinations and have been licensed to practice in your state. Most of us have to agree with the A.M.A., but many of us contend that while all doctors are good, some are better than others, depending on what you want them for, and on your own peculiar tastes and desires. Obviously the A.M.A. cannot rate the abilities of its members as a schoolboy's report card does his.

But the average individual is left without any logical basis upon which to make his choice. And people in general choose their doctor for some strange reasons. One early competitor of mine had a crooked forefinger. He and that finger had a great reputation and a large practice. It was said, and never denied by him to my knowledge, that that finger was peculiarly sensitive; that it would send him vibrations when he passed it over the disease area while examining a patient. He was known by the young wags in town as "the feel doctor." Anyway, many people chose him for that deformed finger.

Some doctors are chosen because they have some gadgetry—an electric shocking machine, a vibrator, being able to make a diagnosis by examining the iris of the eye, or by measuring the "ohms of resistance" in a drop of dried blood which would show so many ohms of cancer, so many of rheumatism and so many of kidney or liver disease. Right today, dozens of employees of a large electronic plant with its own outstanding medical department, travel some miles to patronize a "bloodless surgeon" who, for $200 and four or five days in his "hospital," can "operate" on almost anything without scalpel, retractors or hemostats. He can "cure" gall bladder disease, appendicitis, ulcers or fibroid tumors of the uterus without cutting or leaving a scar. Be it said to his credit that he declines radical mastectomy, that is, complete removal of the breast.

Of course, most executives are neither so ignorant nor so gullible as to be taken in by these eclectics. Yet, I am frequently surprised at the readiness with which otherwise intelligent men and women "fall for" remedial baths of one kind or another, treacle and raisins or honey and vinegar in the diet, not to mention tonics and pills of questionable potency and purpose. They will accept honey and vinegar almost without question, yet neglect or avoid Salk vaccine for themselves and their children. A matter of degree of unpleasantness, perhaps?

Aside from being attracted to a so-called doctor because of fantastic claims of one kind or another, people have other preferences which have little to do with the physician's competence. One of the best surgeons I ever knew was a former naval officer who had the most prolific conversational profanity I have ever heard, except that intimate and highly personal language used by an army mule-skinner in addressing his mules. Yet this skilled and kindly surgeon was adored by longshoremen and dowagers alike, the former because "there was no B.S. about him," the latter because they were shocked and secretly titillated to learn of a new dimension in the use of the English language. To others, of course, he was anathema. They wouldn't have him to "doctor a sick cat." But in choosing another, they may have missed his unquestionably great surgical skill.

Some prefer a doctor who is unctuous and deferential in his manner; others, one who is impeccably dressed and is dignity personified; still others, one who has a penchant for removing the "muciform sac" as so delightfully portrayed in Shaw's *The Doctor's Dilemma.*

These are personal choices to which every individual has a perfect right. But they are still not based on logic. Other things being equal—that is, between several doctors with equal qualifications—these personal preferences are important and can be indulged in.

Most frequently, perhaps, a physician is chosen on the recommendation of some friend, or because he goes to the same church or belongs to the same lodge or club. There is some logic in this method of choice, but it still may have little to do with the man's competence.

SOME LOGICAL WAYS TO CHOOSE YOUR DOCTOR

1. *The County Medical Society* may be helpful within limitations, and especially for checking on some other recommendation. Again, like the American Medical Association, they cannot rate their members, one against the other. They must even be careful concerning race and religion. They can give you:

Locality if you must have someone whose office is in your neighborhood,

Graduates of specific schools if you wish to stick to the good old Crimson or Blue or Maroon and Gold,

Whether or not certified by a specialty board in a certain specialty (certified specialists are described below),

Hospital affiliations are sometimes available at county medical society offices. You may then ask if the hospitals to whose staff the doctor in question has been admitted are accredited by the Joint Commission on Accreditation of Hospitals. If so, it is a recommendation for him. If not, or if he has no hospital affiliations, go slow.

This is not to condemn all doctors who have no hospital affiliation. Many are good. Some are new in the locality and have not yet become well enough acquainted to get an affiliation. But generally speaking, those who have been admitted to the staff, or to visiting privileges by an accredited hospital, have been judged by their peers as competent and ethical, have agreed to abide by the rather strict hospital rules and are willing to participate in the teamwork so essential to good hospital service.

What Is an Accredited Hospital?

Parenthetically, a word about hospital accreditation may not be amiss at this point. The American Medical Association, American Hospital Association, American College of Surgeons, and American College of Physicians have organized and now fully finance a Board of distinguished physicians and hospital administrators to form a separate and independent non-profit corporation to judge the performance and help raise the standards of hospital practice throughout the country. Their examiners visit all hospitals wishing to be accredited to examine their procedures and see if they meet the minimum criteria established by the Board.

Among these criteria, the hospital must have an organized medical staff with duly elected officers and regular meetings at which attendance is required; they must have a records committee whose responsibility it is to see that all patients have complete and accurate records made out by their doctors and nurses, using a standard nomenclature for the names of diseases and treatment procedures; they must have a tissue committee which employs a pathologist to examine tissue removed surgically to aid in the diagnosis and to see if the operation was justified and the accepted procedure followed; they are encouraged to have an admissions committee to see if the patient's admission was justified and necessary and that his hospital stay is not unduly extended.

The findings of these committees are discussed at staff meetings for the good of the patient and in the interests of better hospital practice. Staff members are given a chance to explain any questionable procedures, and if bad practices are found and they persist, that physician may be dropped from staff membership. The Joint Commission may withdraw accreditation if bad practices continue, or if the criteria are not lived up to. Hospitals already accredited are re-examined periodically.

This is one of the most refreshing examples of the way the medical profession polices itself in the best interests of every patient hospitalized. There is naturally some grumbling from hospitals refused accreditation, and a great hue-and-cry from those whose accreditation is withdrawn, even extending to law suits and on one occasion some threatened gunplay in the Commission's Chicago headquarters. However, the Commission has remained firm in upholding and improving hospital practice throughout the country.

Now to get back to the main theme: how the County Medical Society may help you choose your doctor, the above is about all you can expect from them. But even that much is helpful.

2. *Recommendations of Another Physician.* This is by all odds the best way to get a line on a new doctor. If you have a physician friend, even at some distance, he will be helpful. Physicians have ways to check up on other physicians which are not available to those outside the profession. Most state medical societies have a directory listing all licensed physicians in the state, whether or not they are members of the society, and giving certain information about them. In addition, there is the directory of the American Medical Association which lists every licensed physician in the U.S., whether retired or active and whether in private practice, teaching, research, public health, industrial medicine or the military forces.

The information given on each physician is written in a code which means little to the non-medical person, but it lists the date of birth, the school and year graduated, year of licensure, whether in general practice or a specialist, and the scientific societies to which he belongs. Finally, there is the directory of specialists which lists all physicians who have had special training for a specialty board. It, too, is written in an abbreviated code having little meaning to the non-physician.

Besides consulting these directories, your physician friend often has another physician friend in the locality to whom he can telephone for a more personal appraisal or recommendation. Physicians in general have a very keen perception of the quality of the work done by their colleagues. While it is unethical for them to express a derogatory opinion of a fellow physician, they will be glad to steer you in the right direction.

If your company has a medical director, even in a distant city, he is usually glad to perform this advisory function for you and will often do it with thoroughness and objectivity since one of his most important functions is to help the executives of his company keep well.

3. *Other things being equal*, as to qualifications, location, etc., you may now indulge in personal likes and dislikes. You can't get far with a physician you don't like, though one would hope you don't fall in love with a quack. If he's the right one, your doctor will become almost a member of your family—healer, teacher and father confessor. You must feel full confidence in him, remembering that he may be called upon to affect your destinies profoundly. For this latter reason, you may find yourself choosing one physician; your wife, another.

HOW BEST TO USE YOUR DOCTOR

Having picked out a doctor who seems to meet your requirements and is recommended to you by some other physician, make an appointment and call on him, preferably before you have any need for his services. Tell him frankly what you are looking for, who recommended him, what you expect of a doctor. Tell him your circumstances—financial, occupational, and the size of your family. Discuss fees frankly with him and tell him of any accident and sickness insurance coverage you may have. Ask if he makes house calls in emergencies, and if not whether he has an associate who does, or who can be called when he is not available. Ask his hospital affiliations. Ask if he is interested in helping you keep well through periodic health examinations and whether he will send you a reminder on your birthday, or other fixed date, to come in for a check-up. Remember that he is sizing you up, too, and deciding whether he wants to accept the responsibility of taking you as a patient. He has a perfect right to refuse. In fact, any physician can refuse to accept any patient, except that after he has accepted an emergency call, he cannot walk out on the patient until necessary care has been provided.

Having become mutually satisfied with each other, don't hesitate to call your doctor on any and all health questions. Some busy doctors are a little annoyed at needless calls, but when it comes right down to it they would much rather have you call early than when it is too late, and they would much rather provide you with health service than to have you accept the advice of advertisements, the claims of patent medicines, or the guidance of published articles announcing the discovery of some new miracle drug. Should any of these interest you, ask his opinion of it before buying a barrel full! You can certainly tangle things up for your doctor if you are addicted to self-treatment. For example:

One acquaintance of mine, an astute businessman but a medical ignoramus, read somewhere that a rice diet was good for high blood pressure. His highly competent doctor had told him that his blood pressure was slightly elevated, but no more than might be expected for a man of his age, and not to worry about it. Nevertheless, he did, so put himself on a diet of nothing but rice. He got the wrong kind of rice, he had it cooked wrong so that what little vitamins it had were thoroughly cooked out, he stuck it out for four weeks, then called on the doctor. He had lost weight which he needn't have lost, being a slim man anyway. He had the shakes so badly he could hardly unbutton his shirt. His mouth and tongue were sore and there was a rash on his skin. Given supplementary vitamins and put back on a well-balanced diet, he recovered shortly, but his blood pressure remained the same.

Another man's wife was having a bad time with arthritis. Her doctor was treating her properly with one of the cortico-steroids which often relieve the pain but must be carefully watched. She strained her back and thinking, perhaps, to save the cost of another visit to the doctor, her husband had her lie on an electric heating pad. She went to sleep, the medication so lowered her pain threshold that she did not awaken when the pad got too hot. Result: third degree burns which took a long time to heal.

And here cometh lesson number three: Have a good doctor and use him properly and freely. Follow his instructions to the letter. If they are not clear, tell him so and get them straight in your mind. Write them down so you won't forget them day after tomorrow. Nothing so discourages a doctor as to have his instructions ignored. Remember that if the disability is at all serious, or difficult to diagnose, your doctor can work better in the hospital where he has readily available laboratory, X-ray, electrocardiogram and consultation with other doctors if needed.

If the condition is very serious and you are unhappy about what may seem lack of progress, don't hesitate to ask your doctor for a consultation with another doctor, preferably of his own choosing. Rather than being offended, he is often relieved to have you take the initiative. It is usually better to take his advice on choice of consultant. He can judge better than you who is the best man to advise him on this kind of a condition. Also, he probably has consulting specialists with whom he is accustomed to work. They will understand each other better if they are used to working as a team.

When the time comes for your periodic check-up, be sure to tell him everything, occupational strains or stresses, business or domestic worries, anything that is on your mind, whether you think it has a bearing on your health or not. You can trust his discretion. His records are strictly confidential.

A university professor came in to see me one time complaining of sore mouth, bleeding gums, loose teeth and excessive saliva. I had given him his periodic examinations for some time and felt that I knew his history and physical condition pretty well. But I searched high and low in his recent history for a clue to explain his present condition. Was it scurvy due to lack of vitamin C? No, he ate lots of fruit and fresh vegetables. Was it early pernicious anemia with its characteristic sore mouth? No, his red blood cells and hemoglobin were normal. Was it Vincent's angina, a bacterial infection of the mouth? No, smears from the gums examined under the microscope failed to show the characteristic fusiform bacillus. Could it be secondary syphilis? No, his Wasserman had always been negative and still was. I pressed him to try and recall anything that he had done, or anything unusual that had happened. He could think of none.

Finally, I inspected his laboratory where he frequently spent fourteen to sixteen hours a day. No smell of gases or chemicals. Benches with modern impermeable surfaces. No hoods or ventilators but his work did not require them. The old wooden floor was worn and cracked. Wait! What is that sparkle deep in that crack? A diamond? No, it's mercury! And then the mystery was solved! When I asked him about it, he then recalled for the first time that about ten days ago a student had dropped a flask containing nearly a pound of mercury which spilled all over the bench and onto the floor. He and the student spent an hour picking it up as carefully as possible, mainly because of its value. But he didn't think about the cracks in the floor. He was a meteorologist of the old school and not aware of the poisonous nature of mercury vapor. Quantitative measurements showed that the mercury in the floor cracks had evaporated into the air of that small laboratory with no ventilation until it had reached a concentration of something over ten times the toxic limit! He had mercury poisoning which promptly subsided when he moved out of his lab until it was properly cleaned up.

While not many executives work with mercury without knowing its dangers at least, this incident is told to illustrate the fact that occurrences which seem minor to the individual may have much significance from a health standpoint.

Finally, to use your good doctor right, pay his bills as promptly as possible. If it seems more than you can handle as a cash item, tell him so and tell him your plans for paying it over a period of time. He will almost invariably be perfectly satisfied.

HOW TO ABUSE YOUR DOCTOR

Physician-patient relationships when right are delicate and precious to both. Doctors get boiling mad when any third party, such as an insurance representative, or even their county medical society, seem to be interfering with this relationship. Sometimes the patient destroys or impairs that nicely balanced relationship unwittingly. One of these is the way in which the patient goes about:

Changing Doctors. Despite your care and the invaluable suggestions you have just read in choosing a doctor, you may find that you have made a mistake. This is not necessarily a lifetime marriage. The man you have chosen may disappoint you in one way or another. If so, the way to abuse him and probably close his door to you for all time, is just to walk out and go to another doctor, saying nothing to the first doctor. It is much better to tell him frankly the cause of your dissatisfaction, and that for this particular time at least, you feel you should see another doctor, hoping that you may call him again should the occasion arise. Chances are, he is equally unhappy with you and may consider it a good riddance. Anyway, part friends, thank him for all he *has* done. You may want to call him again some day. If you just walk out, saying nothing, he will hear sooner or later that you are going to someone else. Then, if you ever show up again, he doesn't know whose patient you are, or what the other doctor may have done to and for you.

Shopping Around is another way to abuse your doctor. Some people seem to think that medical service is like any other purchase and that they should seek bids for the lowest price of the best quality. Others are suspicious of doctors in general and want verification of the diagnosis or treatment of the first physician. If the condition is serious, involving a threat to life, your desire for verification is quite natural, and your doctor will be the first to appreciate it. Just tell him you'd like someone else's opinion and either tell him whom you have in mind, or ask him to suggest someone. This way, he can share his laboratory, X-ray and electrocardiographic findings with the other doctor, who may find it unnecessary to repeat all those tests.

Sometimes the patient finds the doctor's advice unpalatable and he shops around until he can find someone who will cure him with less inconvenience. He doesn't want to take off thirty pounds, reducing his excessive food intake "makes me weak." So he hears of a "gland doctor" who reassures him and has him come in twice a week for injections of hormones; or he is afraid of a surgical procedure, so he goes to a bloodless healer or has his spine adjusted three times a week.

Your doctor can't have the slightest objection to your desire for a second opinion before undergoing major surgery, or disrupting your business with a prolonged rest cure. Indeed he will welcome it, and will be glad to help you obtain it. But if he learns that you are "shopping around," it is obvious to him that he does not have your complete confidence, and he will have less interest in you than before. And if you decide to go to a quack to have your ulcer cured by pressing on your spinal nerves, or to have your cancer removed with pills and ointments instead of surgery, don't expect him to come a-running some day when your ulcer is hemorrhaging, or to try to remove your cancer surgically after it has spread to other parts of the body.

Many people have little conception of the time, effort and skill the modern doctor uses in reaching a diagnosis. The patient's history must be carefully taken, including family history, past illnesses and injuries, exact duration and symptoms of the present ailment, and some assessment made of the individual's "nervous make-up," that is, his psychological profile. His physical and mental strengths and weaknesses must be assayed, and these matched up with his physical and mental stresses and strains of the past, the present and the probabilities for the future.

Then come the laboratory tests—blood count, including number and kind of white blood cells; number, size, age and hemoglobin content of the red cells; maybe a platelet count and clotting or prothrombin time; maybe blood chemistry which involves delicate quantitative protein and electrolyte chemistry. Next comes the urinalysis upon which to judge kidney function and the presence or absence of abnormal substances such as sugar, albumin and the metallic toxins such as lead.

Next, and often first, the complete physical examination in which the well-trained eye must detect even slight abnormalities of contour, musculo-skeletal and skin abnormalities, abnormalities of the eye, ear, nose, throat, teeth and gums, and often rectum, oesophagus, colon, bladder, bronchial tubes, and vagina; the well-trained ear with the aid of the stethoscope must pick up abnormalities of breath sounds and heart beats; the well-trained fingers must detect tumors or abnormalities of the spleen and liver, and changes in the normal transmission of the spoken voice through the chest wall. Then came the further revelations of the X-ray, electrocardiogram and sometimes the electro-encephalogram by which brain waves are revealed.

Lest all this sound pretty formidable, I hasten to add that out of respect for the patient's pocketbook and his time, much of the doctor's brain-power is spent on deciding what tests he does *not* need. At the same time much of his work may be devoted to "ruling out" the possibility of some obscure condition which might account for your symptoms. Finally, all these findings—history, laboratory tests, physical examination and the X-ray and electrocardiogram—must be fitted together like a jig-saw puzzle before the doctor can give you anything like a definitive diagnosis, and lay out a course of treatment; or, if it is a routine health examination, before he can pronounce you sound or unsound, and if unsound, what to do about it.

Each physician has confidence in his own skill at history taking and physical examining and confidence in his own laboratory or X-ray consultant or cardiologist who reads the delicate tracings made by the micro-electrical waves generated by the rhythmic beat of the heart muscle. Many of them will not accept the findings of another doctor, no matter how good he may be. And this is as it should be. You are *his* responsibility now. He can't take a chance on being careless or inaccurate, or your best interests will not be served. He does not have quite the same interest if he knows you are likely to be "shopping around."

Curbstone, Cocktail or Dinner Party Advice. One of the finest ways to abuse your doctor—nearly all doctors in fact—is to ask for what we call "curbstone" diagnosis and treatment. The average doctor does not wish to be impolite or unkind, so either quips his way out of a direct answer, or just says, "Well, John, I can't really ask you to take off your clothes and let me give you a thorough examination right here. Why don't you see your doctor about it?" But such questions display such abysmal ignorance of the proper and ethical practice of medicine that the doctor is annoyed or disgusted. Some of the things he would like to say are these:

Meeting an acquaintance who is not one of his patients on the street corner, that individual comes up to the doctor saying, "Doc, what shall I do about this lump on my neck?" What the doctor would like to say is, "Go put a rope around your neck and pull it tight!"

Or, "Doc, what's good for indigestion—I've got it something awful." What the "doc" would like to say is, "Stop eating for good!"

Or a dinner partner may say, "Oh, Doctor! I've heard of your wonderful reputation as a brain surgeon. Now I have these terrible headaches. Do you think an operation on my brain would do any good?" What the doctor would like to say is, "Yes, of course. Do let me remove it. It isn't functioning anyway."

Or she says, "My doctor says I have gouty arthritis. Do you think these delicious looking sweetbreads would hurt me?" To which the doctor might like to reply, "Of course not, madam. I notice you seemed to enjoy the sherry and the caviar too. I hope you enjoy an acute attack of gout just as much."

These and a thousand questions like them asked in the most inappropriate places, assail the average doctor many times. The few unethical ones may suggest an early appointment or a careful examination at their office. But mostly, the doctor is just embarrassed. A few uncouth doctors at a dinner party may see in one of these foolish questions an opportunity to be lionized for the evening, whereupon he launches forth on a long and presumably learned dissertation on the subject at hand, blocking all other conversation, much to the consternation of his hostess.

Speaking of lack of social graces, there are few things more distressing to the hostess than to have two or three doctors among her guests, who go into a huddle in a corner and spend the evening discussing medical subjects, ignoring everyone else in the room. Doctors' wives, when entertaining some doctors and their wives, become reconciled to this, but they really try to teach their husbands better manners.

The fact is, no personal medical question can be answered properly "off the cuff."

General questions of public interest and importance are different. The doctor is glad to express himself freely and publicly on such questions as those concerning Salk vaccine, the need for sewer bonds to properly dispose of community sewage, the needs of the community hospital, and the like.

COMPANY DOCTOR, GROUP CLINIC, OR SOLO PRACTITIONER?

In choosing a physician one must often decide between the company medical director and his medical department; a so-called group-clinic such Lahey in Boston, Mayo's in Rochester, Minnesota, Greenbrier, and their counterparts becoming so numerous over the country; and the solo practitioner who practices alone and is probably the nearest approach to the "old fashioned family doctor." There are advantages and disadvantages in each. A wise choice may be easier if we review these briefly.

Company Doctor

Despite the handicap under which the company physician has often labored in the past, I am a believer in his considerable usefulness to the executive. Again, this may reflect some personal bias because of the superb medical department I inherited in the Metropolitan. However, two things are important to remember:

1. The medical director and his staff must be highly competent as will be discussed in the last chapter. Besides medical competence, they must, of course, have strictly confidential records and they must have a full understanding of the stresses, strains and hazards, if any, under which the executive works.

2. They must limit themselves to preventive medicine and often only partial diagnosis. It is not the obligation of management to provide medical care for its executives and other employees, unless

this be done through a separate arrangement such as a health insurance scheme of some kind, often the result of negotiations at the bargaining table. It is the obligation of management to provide as safe and healthful a working environment for all its employees as possible and to make all reasonable efforts to conserve and improve their health. If the medical department finds that the employee has remediable physical defects, or that he is ill and in need of medical care, he will be referred to his own doctor. Thus, the company's medical department will not essay to cure your ulcer or take out your appendix. But they can be trusted to tell you when you need further medical care and why.

With these limitations in mind, there is no doubt that the company medical director, if there is one, and his immediate staff have a more complete knowledge of the stresses and strains under which you may work, of your past occupational history, including successes and frustrations, and of your ambitions and future prospects. They also have the records of your original pre-employment examination, the subsequent periodic examinations and intervening illnesses.

Thus, they can judge how well you are functioning on this job, and whether some change in working habits or conditions is indicated, and they will discuss this with you. This is a great advantage to you and to the company doctor who examines you. Your own physician can only know as much as you may wish to tell him about things at the shop or office. To go back to our meteorology professor, you won't have to remember to tell him about spilling mercury on the wooden floor. This would have been automatically reported to the medical department and you would have been removed from that laboratory until it was thoroughly decontaminated. They will be more fully aware of any hazards under which you work than any other doctor you can find. And they won't jump to conclusions on industrial toxicology as another physician might.

A private physician was treating a female secretary for persistent headaches, lassitude and mild anemia. As she got a little impatient over getting no relief, he asked her to describe in detail the place in which she worked. On learning that the large office was warmed in the California winters by a gas burning floor heater, he jumped to the conclusion that she had "chronic carbon monoxide poisoning" which accounted for her headaches. She promptly reported this to her boss and to her co-workers. It nearly caused a riot. Other girls recalled that they had occasional headaches too, and what was to be done about that heater? If it wasn't fixed, they'd quit. Careful inspection by the industrial hygiene division of the state board of health showed that the heater was properly vented, that it produced very little carbon monoxide anyway, and repeated quantitative tests of the air in the room showed less carbon monoxide than was found on the streets at times. Besides, it is a question whether there is such a thing as "chronic carbon monoxide poisoning."

I am sorry to have to admit that many otherwise good physicians have little knowledge or experience with health hazards common to the place of work. Some years ago a group-insured industry appeared to be having an epidemic of appendicitis in one of its departments. Now appendicitis is not ordinarily considered a contagious disease. Hence, further investigation was indicated. This disclosed the fact that the appendectomies were all among the workers, none in their families. Furthermore, they all worked in one place, the Battery Shop. Careful examination of "the victims" showed that they all had lead poisoning, and the "lead colic" so characteristic of this disease had been mistaken for acute appendicitis by three doctors unknown to each other, but responsible for taking out eight normal appendixes. Introducing proper ventilation in that shop and stopping the common practice of burning old battery casings in a badly vented stove stopped the epidemic!

Repeatedly we see skin eruptions blamed on some harmless material used at work when it is really due to some systemic disorder; asthma, due to pollen in the air, blamed on some peculiar but harmless odor in the work place; deafness blamed on noise in the shop, even though that noise is less in decibels than the noise in ordinary traffic. Most industries, if they have any kind of medical advice at all, are keenly aware of each of their health hazards and have them well controlled. The practicing physician who has the slightest suspicion that his patient's complaint is induced by something connected with his work has only to telephone the plant physician or the personnel officer to have a full report on the matter or a full-scale investigation made promptly.

The disadvantages of going to the company doctor for the periodic health examination and any intervening complaints or worries are, in my opinion, more imaginary than real. Some feel that there is not enough privacy in the company medical department. If so, either the department is not properly managed, or the individual has exaggerated notions about the amount of privacy he needs. It is reassuring to the other employees to see the executives of the company using the medical department. If telephoned beforehand, the medical director will be glad to arrange an appointment which will eliminate waiting.

Some executives feel that they do not want their personal health problems in any company records. They have a perfect right to feel that way and this may be the deciding factor for them. In the well-run medical department, however, all personal records are kept under lock and key, are handled by a carefully selected few who are repeatedly impressed with the confidentiality of all medical matters and who are severely disciplined for the slightest laxity in this respect. An employee's immediate superior, or the personnel department, has a right to know when an employee, including executives, is disabled, about how long the disability will last, something of the seriousness or mildness of the cause, and whether the individual is running into trouble on his present job. The exact diagnosis and previous history, however, is privileged information which cannot be disclosed by the doctor without the employee's consent. If the trouble is serious or progressive, such as cancer, affecting the individual's future usefulness to the company, he can nearly always be persuaded to tell the boss himself, or to permit the doctor to do so.

Some executives feel that their medical department is just a routine medical mill, not intended to care for people of importance. It may well be that they are right. If so, they are justified in having nothing to do with it. But if that is the case, they need a new medical director!

A final disadvantage is that your company may have no medical director. This is bad, even if your company is small, for reasons given in Chapter 10.

The Group Clinic

Many physicians prefer to work in groups, where figuratively at least, several doctors are under one roof, specialists are readily available for consultation, and they all benefit from the common use of the laboratory, X-ray, centralized purchasing and bookkeeping. To many physicians, this type of practice has many advantages. Some of these groups take a special interest in examining and advising executives. And a pretty thorough job they make of it, too. The staff usually consists of highly qualified physicians, including specialists. Some such clinics make a point of conserving the executive's time. Others offer an opportunity for rest and relaxation, interspersed with a series of examinations. Some companies encourage the executive to take advantage of such a service annually by paying the bill for it. This sort of scheme has many obvious advantages.

The disadvantages are:

It is costly, especially if the executive has to travel some distance and be hospitalized.

Some physicians practicing alone complain that the group clinic interferes with the patient's right to have complete free choice of physician since, if consultation is needed, he is automatically referred to a specialist within the group. This does not bother me. The patient has no logical grounds upon which to choose a specialist anyway. As with his original choice of physician, he is much better off to get the recommendations of another physician.

The group clinic examination is thorough but sometimes, in my opinion, unnecessarily so. It may include complete blood chemistry, complete gastro-intestinal X-ray series with barium enema, several other routine X-rays, several electrocardiograms, a basal metabolism or other method of testing thyroid function. Your own doctor, or the company doctor who has your records and history, who does the basic routine physical examination, can tell without taking chances, what special examinations may be indicated in your case, if any, and spare you the time and expense of displaying the wares of the medical profession by doing everything they know how to do. The ordinary, basic routine examination can be done in about an hour's time, including laboratory work, with another fifteen minute session the next day, when the laboratory, X-ray and electrocardiogram reports are in, to discuss the findings with you and suggest anything further you need to do.

Some companies insist that since they are paying for the examination, a report of the findings must be sent the president or the personnel department. This is mentioned only to be condemned. It is in truth an invasion of your privacy. Suppose they find that you have a recurrence of that old venereal disease, or that the female executive, though unmarried, is slightly pregnant? The report should be sent only to your own doctor, or to the company medical director, where it will remain confidential.

Finally, the examining doctors, of which there are often several in a group clinic, know no more about the conditions under which you work than you wish to tell them. Suppose your immediate superior is an unreasonable slave driver with executivitis, driving you to ulcers. Are you going to tell that, especially if the report goes to the president? Suppose your wife is a vixen and you've taken a shine to your secretary. Suppose your travel schedule has become so heavy as to cause a serious rift with your family, but if you don't keep up with it, you'll lose out in the company. Conflicts such as these and many others can cause real illness. They are more common among business executives today than most people realize. You may feel more like telling your family doctor about them. Chances are, the company doctor already knows, or suspects some of these things, since he knows what the job demands are, and he knows full well the "ulcer departments" in your company.

During the regime of one vice president in charge of an important department, the medical director found that eight of the twelve sub-executives in that department had, in a period of five years, developed a varied assortment of disabilities of psychosomatic origin. (See Chapter 7 for psychosomatic disorders.) One had asthma which he had never had before, three had duodenal ulcers and one a stomach ulcer, two had skin rashes and one had so-called mucous colitis. When this vice president retired, they all recovered!

The Solo Practitioner

You may have a family doctor who has known you for years, or you may have carefully selected your physician in a new locality as suggested previously. There is no question but that he can give you unique and valuable services. He knows your strengths and limitations better than anyone else, as well as your past medical history. You should never break such a happy affiilation if you are lucky enough to have it.

Some individuals will travel some distance to have a periodic check-up by their long-time physician, and it's often worth doing. The advantages here are obvious. It should be borne in mind, however, that the medical director of your company will be glad to send your personal physician a full report on your periodic check-up, and on any other findings he may discover when you come in to him for some complaint which seems minor to you. Your personal physician may always feel free to call the company medical director when he is puzzled about any condition he discovers which may arise as a result of your work. He should always advise the company medical department when, in his opinion, you need a change of pace, a vacation or a period of time on disability.

The possible disadvantages of relying entirely on the private physician practicing alone are:

He may have little interest in preventive medicine, being too engrossed with diagnosing and treating sick people. Many, I could almost say most, doctors are this way because their medical school and hospital training is almost exclusively focused on diagnosis and therapy. The number of hours in the medical school curriculum devoted to the teaching of preventive medicine is minimal, to say the least. With many students this small amount of learning is washed off as soon as they pass final examinations on it. With some, however, the small seed of prevention planted in medical school does take root and we find them later in practice exerting a powerful influence in providing their patients with good preventive medicine services.

Your personal physician knows only as much or as little about the stresses and strains of your job as you may wish to give him, as has been mentioned. You can remedy this by "telling all." Carey McCord says that a little bit of every man is worn off onto his job each day. Some jobs are more abrasive than others. Some individuals are more easily abraided than others. It is your doctor's responsibility to see how you are taking it from year to year.

Finally, if you do need the services of a specialist for some special type of examination, such as eyes, complete X-rays of the gastro-intestinal tract, bladder and kidney tests, you will usually have to go to some other building for it on a later appointment. This is not a hardship, merely an inconvenience.

HOW ABOUT THE SPECIALIST?

The true specialist in this country is a physician who has taken from three to five years' additional training, after completing medical school and internship, in some special branch of medicine such as surgery, internal medicine, diseases of the eye, ear, nose and throat, diseases of the heart and blood vessels, of children, of the genito-urinary tract, of the female reproductive system (obstetrics and gynecology) and so forth. There are now some eighteen specialties recognized by the Advisory Council on Medical Specialties of the American Medical Association. The latest, and perhaps the last, is the field of preventive medicine comprising public health, aviation medicine and industrial medicine.

After one or more years of additional didactic training, the would-be specialist spends two to four years as a "resident" in a hospital or other clinical center which has been approved for residency training by the Council on Medical Education of the American Medical Association. Here he is brought along, step-by-step under the exacting tutelage of the "masters" on the staff who literally guide his hand and train his eyes and ears. After this, most boards require a year or two in the actual practice of his specialty, preferably still under the guidance of one of the "masters," after which he writes a thesis based on his actual experience.

Then and then only is he admitted to the examination. The examinations are carefully constructed by the examining boards, lasting at least two days and consisting of a written part and an oral or practical part where he is assigned a patient or two for diagnosis and proposed treatment or is given some other practical problem to work out. The failure rate in these examinations runs from 20 to 30 per cent, so they are far from perfunctory. If successful, he is given a certificate by the board indicating that he is proficient in his specialty.

Later, having earned this certificate, he may or may not be elected to membership in the College or Academy which encompasses his specialty, such as The American College of Surgeons, American College of Physicians, Academy of Pediatrics, Academy of Occupational Medicine and so forth. He is listed in the American Directory of Specialists. Attainment of these honors indicates that he confines his practice solely to his specialty, that he is pledged not to split fees with physicians who refer cases to him, and a number of other high ethical principles.

It is customary among these true specialists not to accept patients unless they are referred by some other physician. This protects them from patients whose real needs lie elsewhere or who do not need special attention at all.

There are many physicians who simply indicate special interest in a certain field. They are so listed in the A.M.A. directory, but they do not necessarily confine their practice to that specialty and they have not necessarily been certified by one of the specialty boards. Many of them are good, but the distinction should be made between them and those who are board certified.

There is little question but what the board certified specialist in this country is one of the best trained physicians the world has ever known. Specialty practice has become more and more popular during the past two generations. Some medical schools report over 70% of their graduates entering a specialty. One cannot but admire these young men who spend four years in college, four years in medical school, one or two years in their internship, and then another three to five years learning their specialty. If to this is added two years' military service and two years to build up a practice, it means the young man is fifteen years out of high school and is in his thirties before he is fully supporting himself and family.

It is a long and exacting discipline, perhaps more so than any other profession. It is necessary, however, lest the medical specialist come to know "more and more about less and less." He must always be fully aware that he is treating the whole patient, not just the eye or the heart or the bladder. That is why, when he starts his graduate studies to prepare for his specialty, he must go back to his original books on anatomy, neurology, physiology and biochemistry to remind him that a disorder in one organ may upset many others that are interrelated, notably the nervous system.

WHAT OF THE CULTS?

There are so many ways of simulating the healing arts and sciences that they cannot be listed or catalogued here. Suffice it to say that they are all unorthodox in the eyes of those who have spent ten to fifteen years in orthodox learning. Fortunately, they are not so numerous now as they were two generations ago, thanks to the medical practice acts in the various states, and the sound criteria for acquiring medical competence set up by the medical profession itself. Near the turn of the century, Dr. Abraham Flexner made a study of medical schools in this country and issued a courageous report to the Carnegie Foundation. He found over three hundred schools giving the M.D. degree, most of them proprietary, many little more than diploma mills. It was largely through the courageous and relentless work of the Council on Medical Education and Hospitals of the American Medical Association, first led by the late Dr. Ray Lyman Wilbur, that this situation was remedied. Today, there are but eighty-two medical schools in this country, all rated as Class A, all inspected periodically by impartial representatives of the Council, and all meeting the strict criteria recommended by the Flexner report and upgraded since.

Nevertheless, I am not one to uphold orthodoxy just for its own sake. There is no doubt that stubborn adherence to orthodoxy has sometimes been a stumbling block to progress in the medical profession. For example, John Hunter, despite his notable discoveries in the 18th century, was berated by the medical profession of London for his unorthodox views; Louis Pasteur, who as a mere chemist could not be expected to be taken seriously by the French medical profession; Charles Darwin, whose new theories on the evolution of the species set off a great controversy in medical, ecclesiastical and lay circles; William Jenner, a student of John Hunter's, who discovered vaccination against smallpox, has been resisted by some for over a hundred years; and many others. To the non-medical person, this may be an indication of stubborn stuffiness on the part of organized medicine. Indeed, that's just what it is in many instances.

On the other hand, there is a certain virtue in this reluctance to accept new and revolutionary ideas by the majority of the medical profession. It means that organized medicine, in the interests of the public, will not be stampeded hither and yon by the many unorthodox theories brought forth almost daily by the armchair philosophers. These theories are often the product of what David Starr Jordan called "armchair reasoning," where the theorist is too lazy or too ignorant to test his conclusions in the laboratory or the field, or to describe his experiments, if any, in detail and encourage others to verify his conclusions by using the same meticulous protocols. Indeed, when the exacting methods of good scientific experimentation are followed, the medical profession has been surprisingly quick to accept new discoveries, especially in recent years—witness the terrific demand for penicillin, streptomycin and for Salk vaccine so quickly after their value had been proved beyond a doubt.

Faith Healing

As one looks back over the history of medicine, there is even some evidence that at least some of the cultist theories eventually had a beneficial effect on medical orthodoxy. Among the oldest examples is that of "faith healing," originating centuries ago in the tribal medicine man and evolving gradually to the present day in the healing beliefs of the Christian Science Church and appearing from time to time in other religions, such as the "laying on of hands" by certain Protestant beliefs, and the various healing shrines of the Catholics, such as Lourdes. Orthodox medicine has gradually absorbed and given some scientific credence to some of these beliefs through psychiatry. Among examples of this is the credence now given to the enormous power of suggestion, and the gradually emerging respectability of hypnosis.

Nevertheless, some so-called faith healers are nothing less than charlatans. They prey upon, rather than pray for, the ignorant and the gullible. No good physician will discount the value of prayer. We often gladly share the credit for recovery with our brethren of the cloth. But no good physician will condone the healer of any faith who obstructs the benefits of modern medicine while his patient neglects the early cancer, the relief of diabetes, the remediable birth defects and the failing but recoverable heart.

Osteopathy No Longer a Cult?

Had Andrew Taylor Still brought his bag of bones into Bellevue Hospital today, instead of exploiting it under the name of osteopathy in Kirksville, Missouri, three generations ago, we in medicine would most surely have called him a crackpot, as we still do. Nevertheless, the effectiveness of his "laying on of hands" in relieving the symptoms of some people gave us pause for thought. Perhaps it stimulated us to pay more attention to the now unquestioned value of passive massage and the now invaluable field of physiotherapy in the rehabilitation of some of the sick and injured. Although his theories were purely the product of "armchair reasoning," and even yet have never been proved by scientific methods, they led to the gradual elevation of the cult of osteopathy until today several osteopathic schools approach equality with some of the medical schools, and there is talk of amalgamating the American Osteopathic Association with the American Medical Association.

Still's theory, later paraphased and simplified by the chiropractors, was that the flow of life and health reached all parts of the body through the nerve system, especially as the greater nerves emerged from the spinal cord through the natural openings between the vertebrae of the spinal column. Maladjustment of the vertebrae, the causes of which were not very specific, caused interference with normal transmission of either the nerve impulses or the circulation—sometimes one, again the other, and thus disrupted the normal health of that portion of the body supplied by that nerve. By pushing, pulling or otherwise manipulating the maladjusted vertebrae back into place, health was restored to the sick parts. This usually required several visits at so much per, and was likely to recur, requiring another series of treatments. Today, many graduates of the better schools of osteopathy pay little attention to Still's original tenets.

Homeopathy an Outworn Cult?

Another armchair medical philosopher was "Doctor" Samuel Hahnemann, the founder of homeopathy, who believed that "similia similibus curantur," (like cures like). To oversimplify his theories: if you had a stomach ache *exactly* like the stomach ache caused by eating green apples, then essence of green apples diluted with water or alcohol to 1 part in a million, or even 100 million (as the high potency enthusiasts claimed) and given in 2 or 3 drop doses further diluted in half a glass of water (it was never a full glass), and given in teaspoonful doses every 15 to 30 minutes, would cure that stomach ache.

Hahnemann and his followers claimed some remarkable results and their patients became quite devoted to them. It is to be noted, however, that the homeopathic doctor usually stayed with the patient for the first two or three teaspoonfuls, often exuding confidence, comfort and reassurance. When he left, one of the family was delegated to sit up all night if necessary administering the teaspoonful faithfully as prescribed. That much sympathetic and kindly attention would, in my opinion, even today cure a large proportion of the acute minor ills of mankind.

Nevertheless, the gentle ministrations of Hahnemann and his followers brought out the fact that many people feared and avoided the overdosage of strong medicine then in vogue among the "allopaths," including purging, blood letting, mercury and arsenicals, and even the springtime tonic of asafetida and sulphur and molasses.

Orthodox medicine began to have another look at its medicinal armamentarium, leading to the era of Sir William Osler when drug therapy commenced to be calibrated and the action of the drug aimed at the actual pathology of the cells. By that time, thanks to Virchow and the school of cellular pathology, the actual cause of many illnesses could be demonstrated.

To give credit where it is due, it should be noted with respect to these two cults, osteopathy and homeopathy, as the standards of medical education were raised, so too were the standards raised by their respective schools. Right from the start of homeopathy, the medical student got the benefit of all the teaching given in the orthodox medical schools, *plus* the teaching of homeopathic medication. Not during Still's day, but more frequently in recent years, some of the osteopathic medical schools have the same premedical requirements, approximately the same number of hours in the medical sciences, *plus* the teaching of osteopathic manipulation. At no time were the homeopathic schools giving any less training to their students. Of late, the best of the osteopathic schools are reaching that same standard.

And that's what it comes down to. If you have any question about the safety, effectiveness and usefulness of any of the cultists, inquire into the amount of training they get. We in medicine think it takes a minimum of seven or eight years before the student can be trusted to diagnose and treat patients on his own, and even then we like him to have one or two more years under close surveillance in a good hospital before he is out on his own.

Chiropractic healing was an offshoot of osteopathy founded by Daniel Palmer, a former student of Still's. Chiropractors concentrate on manipulation of the spine, believing that illness of almost any part of the body is caused by pressure on the nerves as they emerge from the spinal column. By pressing on these nerves and the surrounding bony foramina in the spinal column, they believe they restore normal circulation and normal transmission of the nerve impulses, thus allowing health to return to the body. They are not licensed in all states. Those who are licensed must confine their practice to chiropractic, avoiding surgery, obstetrics and all but limited medication. Their training seldom exceeds two years, and the curriculum often includes salesmanship, accounting and bill collecting, propaganda and advertising.

Chiropody or *Podiatry* is often confused with chiropractic, but they mean the treatment of the feet. There is little doubt that the human foot has suffered from civilization. Ill-fitting shoes, sometimes from infancy; the impact of city pavements; long hours of standing; and the lack of proper exercise have all taken their toll on the foot. When this is combined with impaired circulation as we get older, and especially in rather advanced cases of hardening of the arteries and of diabetes, even minor abrasions on the feet may present serious complications.

The orthodox physician rarely paid much attention to the ills of the flat footed and the foot weary. Thus, this minor but important specialty now called podiatry grew up and there are several schools giving two or three year courses and turning out practitioners who are generally trustworthy, who abide by their limitations and do much for the footsore and weary by removing calluses, corns, and plantar warts, treating bunions and attempting to restore normal balance to the abused and decrepit foot. Many of them are on the staffs of teaching hospitals where the medical staff members ask them to attend the needs of the diabetic and arteriosclerotic. In fact, if we take literally the oft repeated cry, "Doctor, my feet are killing me," they save many a life!

Others. There are a host of other cultists who practice one or another forms of the healing arts: naturopaths, bloodless healers, some masseurs, high colonic irrigation, ruptures and piles cured without the knife. Some of them advertise their wizardry with electrical devices, others push their patent medicines comprising a "secret formula" or containing the ingredients "all doctors use." Perhaps the most harmful are those who claim to have a cure for cancer. They entice the gullible to try their remedy, or come to their clinic, losing precious time when the cancer might have been removed completely by surgery or radiation or a combination of both. Perhaps the following suggestions will be helpful in either avoiding them, or if you wish to give them a trial, proceeding with caution:

Suggestions for Avoiding Harm by Cultists

1. Have nothing to do with any kind of healer who guarantees a cure. Only the knave or the fool will do this. Even the best qualified physician treating the simplest malady knows that he treats and God cures. The diagnosis may be wrong, the treatment wrong, or God is looking elsewhere.

2. Bear in mind that much of what goes on in the human body in health as well as disease is still a mystery. The best of training in the structure and functioning of the body and mind is none too good to be entrusted with this precious possession of yours. It is the only body and mind you will ever have. Let no charlatan fool with it!

3. It does take a long time to learn and utilize properly what *is* now known about health and disease and therapy. If you are tempted by a healer who does not have the M.D. degree, find out how much formal training he has had in the study of his particular brand of healing. Generally speaking, the man with the most training, plus continued learning experience, is the best man to go to if you are sick or injured.

It is my firm conviction that no healer with less than seven years' intensive training in an accredited medical or osteopathic school should be entrusted with the treatment of a fracture, pneumonia, cancer, heart disease or other serious disease, or with major surgery.

4. Take your doctor into your confidence and tell him that you would like to give this or that cultist a try. Unless the cultist is an out-and-out faker, your doctor won't object, even though he doesn't approve. Report back to him on the results you are getting from time to time.

5. Finally, remember that in most states almost anyone may use the title "Doctor." It does not mean that he is a doctor of medicine with the M.D. degree from an accredited medical school. On the other hand, it is against the law in most states to practice medicine without a license to do so. Your cultist may be licensed to practice chiropractic or naturopathy or bloodless healing, but he is restricted to that particular method. Find out what kind of a license he has and what its restrictions are. This may be obtained from the State Board of Medical Examiners, the State Board of Licensure, or whatever it may be called in your state. Your doctor can tell you.

CONCLUSION

In conclusion, let me be as fair and objective as possible with the eclectic methods of healing and to those who really do find relief at the hands of some cultists.

There can be no doubt that many people suffer from functional disorders, that is those in which no organic changes can be found by the best of doctors to account for the symptoms. And their number is legion. These are the vague, but often disabling aches and pains, worries and sorrows which afflict most of us at one time or another to a greater or lesser degree. There can be no doubt that some people are more easily disabled than others. That is not a reason to condemn them. It's the way they are built. For example:

It so happened that during the first world war, we had in our base hospital in France two soldiers in the same ward each of whom had to have a leg amputated just above the knee. Both surgical procedures were identical and were done by the same surgical team. Both had the same nursing and ward attendants. One complained from the moment he came out of the anesthetic. He had great pain in the foot that was gone; he would not lie still but disarranged his dressings several times a day; he screamed when the dressings were changed; he could not eat the food; and worst of all, he could not seem to reconcile himself to a life on one leg. He claimed to see no reason for living. He was badly disabled and remained so even through the convalescent hospital and back to the states to have an artificial limb fitted. After discharge he did not work for years.

The other lad, with exactly the same disability, was cheerful from the moment he awoke minus his leg in the ward. He joshed his ward mates, kidded the nurses, insisted on a crutch at the earliest possible moment so that he could get to the bath room, was much interested in the kind of "wooden leg" he was going to have and wanted to have it now so the boys could write their names on it. He had a good mechanical leg and was working at a good job many months before the other boy would even try to learn to use his artificial leg.

Now this is not to say that the first boy was not disabled. Imaginary it might have been, and this concept often tries the patience of the doctors and nurses. But he was in travail. He was sick in mind and body. He would literally have starved before he finally went to work if no one had cared for him. He was just "built that way" with a combination of poor attitudes, a "sensitive nervous system" and a marked degree of immaturity and emotional instability. Interestingly enough, he did finally "grow up" and became quite a useful citizen when he learned to overcome his travail.

My point here is that a pain is a pain. Another person can't see it or feel it, but it's there as far as the sufferer is concerned. If a faith healer, a masseur, a chiropractor or other cultist can relieve that pain, more power to him, say I. What if he does do it by the power of suggestion, or by the laying on of hands, or the Coué system by repeating, "I am better every day in every way," or by the mere encouragement of holding a hand and soothing a fevered brow, let us be thankful that suffering is relieved. Orthodox doctors may not endorse the method used, but few will object to seeing the elimination of the pain and the relief of disability, providing the method used does no harm.

That is why it is wise to check with your regular doctor from time to time while patronizing a cultist. We have known of individuals with tuberculosis of the spine whose spines were broken by an ignorant "healer" using forceful manipulation. We have seen an acute neuritis or bursitis greatly aggravated by an insufficiently trained manipulator. Saddest of all are those with progressive disease, such as cancer or tuberculosis, who waste precious time with some healer's incantations, or medications. At the same time, with the exception of those who are manifest fakers, ruthlessly playing on human ignorance and gullibility, some of these eclectic theories may have been of some benefit to orthodox medicine over the years. We have always known that a strong religious faith sustains and comforts the sick and dying. We are learning much about the power of suggestion and the legitimate uses of various forms of hypnosis.

As a rather ribald example of the power of suggestion, we could nearly always send a freshman medical student scuttling into the eye clinic if three or four upperclassmen would buttonhole him in the corridors, look intently into his eyes and say, "I thought so, you are a bit cross-eyed."

There is an old story which also illustrates the power of suggestion: The elderly mother was carried to the hospital for an emergency appendectomy which went smoothly. On the second day, following routine orders, the nurse got her out of bed to take a step or two. She insisted that she could not walk. The nurse said, "I know, that's what they all say. Come on now, take my hand." Each day she took a few more steps and finally walked to the car to be taken home. The son, amazed to see her so well called the surgeon to thank him. "Doctor," he said, "you have performed a miracle!" "Oh," said the doctor, "it was really nothing, just a routine appendectomy." "But, doctor," insisted the son, "you don't understand. Mother hasn't walked for three years!" The power of suggestion lies in the fact that the nurse had no question in her mind but that the patient could walk and she literally forced her to do so. That faith and confidence was transmitted to the patient.

So the cultists are not *all* bad. But proceed with caution. Most of them are suspect.

CHAPTER
3
TRICKS OF THE FOREBRAIN

Now that we have seen that the only occupational disease to which the executive is prone to executivitis, and that it may be prevented and cured with the help of a well-selected doctor who is used properly; and since we have taken a peek into some of the underlying psychological causes which may interfere with the best of health, let us probe a little deeper into these interferences.

We all have one piece of apparatus in our bodies which may trip us up. No, it is not the sex organs, though they will bear watching. They too will be influenced to a large extent by the functioning of this trickster. It is the forebrain.

WHAT IS THE FOREBRAIN?

The forebrain is that large mass of brain material which comprises the frontal lobes and their supporting brain tissue, the size and complexity of which distinguish man from the lower animals. Apes come the closest to man in the size of their forebrain, though it is still much smaller. Lower animals, such as chickens and worms, have practically none. Herein lies memory, the ability to develop ideas based on some kind of reasoning, the ability to associate one experience with another, and a great variety of functions unique to man. It is a great mass of nerve fibers, insulated one from another, but connected in innumerable ways with one another and with the midbrain, the hind brain and the spinal cord.

So intricate are these connections, and so numerous, that no one has ever figured them all out. Suffice it to say that the human child learns, with the help of this intricate apparatus, more in the first two years of life than could possibly be taught him as one would teach new tricks to a performing dog. It is the prize possession of *homo sapiens,* such as no other living thing has. It has variously been called the seat of the soul, the spirit, the personality and the source of civilization. Naturally, the early anatomists considered it essential to life.

SCRAMBLED BRAINS?

Some years ago, a man was brought into the clinic at a medical school. He had committed an error not uncommon with miners. They seldom do it more than once! He had rammed his crowbar down a drill-hole in the rock, at the bottom of which was an undischarged load of dynamite. By some freak it did not blow his head off, but the crowbar was driven through his eye socket and the handle emerged through the top of his skull. Yet here he was alive, able to walk, talk, and otherwise act normal! He became a great pet of the students and the professors, the latter using him for demonstration before medical classes from time to time. Eventually he died of natural causes and it is said that his skull is still preserved in the medical school museum.

We know now that at least not all of the forebrain is essential to life. It was not until many years later that we learned through the brilliant work of Dr. John Fulton and his followers at Yale, working with some of the great apes, that with certain incurable cases of insanity, a lobotomy could be performed. This consisted of making several slices through the frontal lobes of the brain, thus presumably disrupting certain faulty "circuits" which had developed, either causing, or resulting in, the insanity. To be sure, these people were not very productive thereafter, living more as vegetables, but most of them retained the power of speech and locomotion, and no longer required confinement for their mental disability.

HOW BEST TO LIVE WITH THE FOREBRAIN INTACT?

So, we see that it is possible to live without an intact forebrain. The question is how best to live, as most of us fortunately do, with the forebrain intact? How may we take full advantage of this amazing piece of apparatus, use it to help us as it was meant to do, and learn to avoid or at least recognize some of the dismaying tricks it may play on us.

This brings us into the field of psychosomatic medicine—"psycho" meaning the mind, and "soma" meaning the body; in other words, the effect of mind over matter so far as the body is concerned. This is no place for a book-length discussion of how emotional disturbances may cause demonstrable physical disturbances. Suffice it to say that they do, and they are nothing to be ashamed of. Too many people assuming a sophistication they do not possess say in a derogatory tone, "Oh, that headache of yours is all psychosomatic," implying that it is either self-willed, or imaginary. That's not so. A psychosomatic ailment is not imaginary. It is a real disability, and most doctors treat it as such. It may be self-willed, but so is a broken leg sometimes, and the reasons for a subconscious wish for a disability are deep-seated and often hard to accept by the victim.

HOW ABOUT ANIMALS?

First, let us see what disturbances of the forebrain, where emotions largely originate, will do to animals. To be sure, many higher-type animals seem to have emotions, especially pets of humans, but in the main they are less discernible than in humans.

In some of the early studies on the causes of arteriosclerosis or "hardening of the arteries" in humans, few animals were found naturally subject to this condition. It could be produced only by some artificial means, such as surgery or drugs.

In an experiment in Russia, which might not meet the enthusiastic approval of the SPCA here, a male monkey was confined in a cage and a rival male turned loose to seek his pleasure among his harem of females, all within plain sight of the caged monkey. Within the confines of his cage, he showed every evidence of displeasure and frustration! He screamed expletives at his rival, hurled himself at the bars, and in monkey language promised death and destruction to his enemy. The latter was not impressed, but went on his way rejoicing with the females. The caged monkey's blood pressure rose markedly, as might be expected, but subsided when his rival was removed from sight.

As time went on, however, and in the course of a few weeks of this treatment, the caged monkey developed a permanent elevation of blood pressure and evidence of hardening and thickening of the arteries. When he came to autopsy, the arteries were permanently thickened and hardened. There was actual enlargement of the arterial wall, narrowing of the lumen, and a resulting reduction of blood supply in the arteries of the heart and the other organs and muscles. He was a likely victim of heart attack or apoplexy or kidney disease. Of course, the simple lesson here for human males is: If your wife is inclined to commit indiscretions with other men, don't stand where you can see her—it may give you high blood pressure.

But more important, for all human beings, this seems to demonstrate that even in the absences of infection, or drug or chemical poisoning, or extremes of diet, long continued emotional strain will actually produce demonstrable pathology in otherwise normal body cells, in this case, the cells lining the arteries. It would do the human prototype of this kind of a monkey (and with a little stretch of the imagination, you will recognize many such) little good to tell him that his high blood pressure is psychosomatic.

In another experiment of great value to humans, a tiny electrode carrying an infinitesimal electric current was placed in a certain spot in a monkey's brain. Placed in other spots, it had no effect, so minute was the electrical stimulation. In six weeks, almost to the day, the monkey developed a stomach ulcer. It takes but little imagination to replace the monkey with a human being, and the electrode with a constant worry, fear, frustration or other strain which exists only in the brain, to understand why a persistent upsetting emotion can cause stomach ulcer. It is another proof that emotional disturbances will actually cause illness which is demonstrable in pathology in the body tissues. This is not to say that *all* ulcers of the stomach and duodenum are due to emotional causes, but only that *some* of them are.

We once had a pet poodle, who like "The Dog That Wouldn't Be," thought she was people. We did not disillusion her. When our domestic tranquility was interrupted by a journey on which we could not take her, she had perforce to go to the very good boarding kennel. There, she told us in no mistakable terms she was "treated like a dog" and didn't like it one bit. It got so that if we even got to talking about a trip together without her, she would go into a blue funk days before our departure. And when we brought out the bags and commenced to pack, she would vomit—always on the rug!

Now she was a strong little dog with a cast-iron stomach, judging from the variety of things she relished without the slightest indigestion. We were certain that this vomiting was not caused by any dietary indiscretion or any infection. What did cause it was dislike of our absence and the kennels—worry, fear, protest and frustration, psychic rather than somatic illness. So you see, this can happen even to a dog.

Teachers, school nurses and pediatricians frequently encounter vomiting in young children sent to school for the first time. There is nothing wrong with them physically, as the doctor often says. They're just homesick and don't want to leave mamma and go to school. Again, this is an emotional upset that shows itself in physical manifestations.

LIKEWISE BIG STRONG HE-MEN

Enough about the brain waves of monkeys, dogs and children —what about men? Yes, there are signs all about us that even big strong he-men are susceptible to the same tricks which may be played on them by the forebrain. The attending physician at one of the large stock exchanges tells me that his dispensary is much more popular during a period of market depression. Colds, coughs, wheezes, indigestions and rheumatics seem more common when men are under strain and apprehension. A while ago a study was made of C.P.A.'s specializing on income tax reports. Though limited to a certain age-group and geographic area, this study seemed to show a higher incidence of coronary attacks and of peptic ulcers during that frantic season just preceding the dead line for filing returns.

The well-trained and observing company doctor gives us many examples of illnesses triggered by work situations, some of which were referred to in the previous chapter. Among themselves, these specialists in industrial medicine refer to the "ulcer departments" within their respective companies and to the executives, who are "ulcer givers" and those who are "ulcer getters." Thrice blest are those increasing numbers of medical directors who can, and do, proudly boast that their top executives understand the vicissitudes of the work environment, the frailties of human nature, and the fact that one of their primary responsibilities is to "get better than average work out of average people" without doing them harm. Indeed, this is the modern, often younger type of executive who has escaped or cured executivitis, and their number is increasing.

A GOOD TRICKSTER

It should be plain then, that the brain, especially the forebrain, is probably the most priceless endowment of the human. Tricks it may play on us from time to time, but these are not all bad. Those that are upsetting are to be expected and they will do no great harm, providing we recognize them for what they are and learn to adjust to them, just as we have, over the centuries, learned to walk upright. The brain is what makes us what we are. Here lies the seat of personality, of character, memory, inventiveness, artistry and the progress of civilization as we have known it.

Brain power often transcends serious physical handicaps as in Milton's blindness, Franklin D. Roosevelt's paralysis, Steinmetz's deformed spine, and the many who have become famous despite serious tuberculosis as brought out in the book, *Conquerors of Fate,* by the famous, and one-time tuberculous, lung specialist,

J. A. Myers. And brain power can be developed throughout life, perhaps to an even greater extent than any other function of the body. We who are in business or the professions often wish that the thousands of indifferent college students over-running the "halls of ivy" today could realize that a formal college education is far less important from the standpoint of what they learn than from the standpoint of learning how to learn. Few attainments are more valuable to the individual than the ability to learn throughout life.

INFINITE HUMAN VARIATIONS

There is wide variation in individuals, especially in their nervous systems, meaning the brain and all its connections. These are probably largely hereditary, although, as with nearly all brain functions, they can be developed enormously once the "tendency" is detected. The great symphony conductors and composers, for example, live in a different world of hearing than do those who are tone deaf. They actually hear a wider range of sounds on the musical scale and a greater combination of sounds than do average people. The great painters have an entirely different "feel" for colors and their combinations than do average individuals. Some people's taste-buds are much more sensitive than others'. From the constructive standpoint they may develop this proclivity into becoming tea, coffee or wine tasters, or great chefs, or merely the enjoyable avocation of being gourmets. From the destructive standpoint they may just become neurotically fussy about their food. Some folks have a much lower pain threshold than others, becoming really seriously disabled with a minor degree of pain, while others can stand the dentist's drill without a grimace and without novocaine.

Incidentally, and aside for the moment, women in general stand pain better than men, contrary to the popular belief. This is in spite of the fact that there is some evidence that their pain threshold in general is lower than that of men; that is, they feel slighter degrees of pain more acutely. But they stand it better.

In the summer of 1916 we were giving smallpox vaccine to a

regiment of national guardsmen before they left for the Mexican border. The men stood in line, two hundred at a time, awaiting the "operation," then stood in line again to let the scarified area dry before putting on a light dressing. None fainted while having a bit of skin of the arm scraped with a scalpel, an antiquated technique which gives the modern doctor the shudders. But while standing in line, either before or after, about twenty out of every two hundred "keeled over" in a faint. The interesting phenomenon was that if the first fainter happened to be near the front of the line, in sight of all the others, eight or ten more back of him would promptly fall over. Indeed, they went down almost like a row of dominoes!

A few years later I had occasion to vaccinate several hundred teen-age girls in a school. Though they stood in line in equal numbers and for about the same length of time, not one of them fainted! Big husky he-men, hey? But too many with tricky forebrains.

The interesting sequel to this story is that this same regiment of horse-drawn artillery, in less than eighteen months, was part of the Rainbow Division of the American Expeditionary Forces in France, and many of these very same men who fainted at the sight of vaccination were cited for acts of great bravery. It was the way they *felt* about the vaccination. And how they felt about vaccination originated in their forebrain. The trickster!

As I look back, I fear too many of these really sturdy fellows who fainted felt guilty about it, and of course their guilt was compounded by the unrestrained jeers of their fellows, including some members of the medical detachment, who should have known better. These tricks of the forebrain are nothing to be ashamed of. More often than not, they just can't be helped. But we can recognize them for what they are, and not be unduly upset by them.

Well, we were talking about the great variation in different persons in the way their brain and nervous system reacts to certain stimuli. This same variation applies to tricks of the forebrain. Some seem born with a "bovine placidity." Nothing upsets them unduly.

Worries are just not their dish. They accept and seem to make the best of their fortune, good or ill. How fortunate they really are! Others are nervous, highstrung, jittery and jumpy. Are they all entirely unfortunate? Well, let's think twice before answering that.

A genius is not always the happiest person in the world. He or she is not always easy to live with. They are often beset with more than their fair share of the tricks of the forebrain. Nevertheless, they often accomplish what others thought impossible. You see, these tricks of the forebrain are not always destructive or harmful. As often as not, they are helpful to an uncanny degree. They permit, or produce, a freer association of ideas. They often enable the mind of the genius to reach far back into his subconscious to an almost forgotten experience or observation which is related to, and sheds some light on, a problem at hand. They may engender a rebellious disregard for orthodoxy, and thus enable the mind to take an entirely new approach toward solving a problem.

Who but one with the mind of an Edison could have thought of linking the heat produced by a material resistant to an electrical current, to the production of light? We can probably safely surmise that he never read it in a textbook on electrical engineering, nor would he have learned it from the professor if he had gone to college instead of leaving school to be a peanut butcher on a train. These tricks of the forebrain often bring questions to the mind that no one has ever thought of asking before. And when they are linked with ambition and drive, there comes an overpowering desire to find the answer to such unorthodox questions.

The plain fact is that the human mind en masse does not usually care to be disturbed by troublesome questions which require effort to answer. Almost from the beginnings of man, the most popular mental attitude has been. "My mind is made up: don't disturb me with the facts." There is the legend of Giordano Bruno, whose fellow priests became disturbed over the question, "How many teeth has a horse?" The books of the day were searched and there was much speculation without finding the answer. When Bruno suggested catching a horse and counting his teeth, he was found guilty of heresy and lack of faith in the good books, and burned at the stake.

So, we see that many of the tricks of the forebrain are good, even if disturbing. Today, they may not lead to burning at the stake, but they may even yet cause ostracism or persecution by the masses who incline toward bovine placidity. More important, if not recognized for what they are and dealt with calmly and sensibly, as any less personal problem would be dealt with, they are capable of causing real illness and pathological changes in the body cells.

DETECTING THE TRICKSTER

Dealing with these tricks sensibly may simply consist of recognition. Often that suffices. You say to yourself, "Damn it! One of those fierce headaches is coming on again." Assuming that your doctor has made a careful search for the cause of these headaches and has found nothing organic to account for them, you will probably find that they are usually connected with some stressful situation in the office or the home.

Recent studies at Cornell have shown that over 90 per cent of recurrent headaches are associated with some kind of stress, usually an emotional upset, which causes the blood vessels in certain areas of the brain either to constrict or dilate, thus producing the headache. With this comes a tensing of the muscles, especially the neck and face. Less than 10 per cent of these recurrent headaches, so troublesome and even disabling, have anything to do with eye strain, blood pressure, digestive upsets or other organic changes. These researchers have even been able to bring on a headache by inducing the patient to talk about some unpleasant subject affecting his personal or business life which has been troubling him for some time. By identifying the subject or the situation which brings on the headache, the patients have been greatly helped either by setting about to correct the problem or avoiding the situations which bring on the headache.

So, you say to yourself, "All right, so what. I can't run this business without occasional stresses or knotty problems. I've always been able to lick them in due time, or I wouldn't be where I am. This one is now licked, or about to be. Maybe it's worth a little time off for a headache." Get out of the office and take a walk, go home and lie down, go to the club and read the *Police Gazette*, take an aspirin, take in a movie, or go to the races. You'll soon forget it, and you'll be fit as a fiddle next morning.

If, on the other hand, you haven't been to the doctor and you're afraid it may be a brain tumor like the one that killed Uncle Ned, or that you're losing your eyesight, or it may be migraine like Aunt Tillie had, or that it's due to high blood pressure and you may be subject to a stroke like your father had, or a myriad of other fears such as only ignorance of the truth can breed—you're in trouble!

If you think to yourself, "God, this job is killing me. I'm really too sick to work this hard. I can't stand it much longer," etc., etc., then the trickster has really got you. One fear leads to another. You may be in for a real disability. You're not in a position to recognize it for what it is: one of those rough spots in every day life for the busy executive, and for that matter, everyone else. Why blow your top? What makes one feel that way?

WHAT DO YOUR FEELINGS DO TO YOU?

We have seen that what made the soldiers faint while awaiting vaccination was how they *felt* about it. So it is with your job as an executive or a future executive. What it does to you depends on how you *feel* about it. Just as surely as one man's meat is another man's poison, so likewise heavy and increasing responsibilities are a joyous challenge for one man, and an overwhelming burden for another. That's the way each man feels about it.

It's an old adage in psychiatry that you can't hide your feelings. You may submerge them for a while, but sooner or later they will show themselves in one way or another. Usually these submerged emotions show up in unpleasant ways such as undue irritability, indigestion, headaches, skin rashes or excesses in eating or drinking.

Many years ago, the chancellor of a great university, himself a physician and a remarkably able educator and administrator, told me he had decided as a young man that emotions were what got most people into trouble, and that he had determined to avoid emotions in his life just as nearly as possible. This statement from so great a man astonished me. I had thought we had outgrown that kind of Puritanism. But as I have thought back upon it, I must admit that what success he had in subduing his emotions worked well for him, for he was a truly great man.

As I study his amazing career more carefully, however, I'm inclined to think that what he really meant was that he did not let his emotions too greatly influence his behavior. He often spoke bluntly, but not in anger. He faced many highly critical situations, but never showed fear. He had good reason to condemn many rascals who crossed his path, but never showed hate.

The point is, a man or woman cannot live without emotions. They are generated in that priceless heritage, the forebrain, and are there for a purpose. They are all to the good. They should be recognized as such—the constructive ones such as love encouraged, the destructive ones such as hate discouraged—as far as possible. Nevertheless, the world is full of rascals and life of vicissitudes. So, you may ask, what is wrong with getting a good hate on once in a while? It brightens the eye, clears the lungs and cures biliousness. You may cite me the old lady, who when asked how she attained such a ripe old age said, "I takes sides and gits mad."

There's something to that argument and I won't deny it. However, behavior controlled by emotions instead of cool reasoning is a luxury not often permitted executives in their business dealings. Usually, it will throw them off balance and do harm where it was not intended. If you must "get a good hate on," express yourself to a confidant and get it out of your system. Or write the rascal a scathing letter, but be sure to send it to your legal counsel, not the hated one. Many seemingly good executives are said to be "hot tempered," that is, quick to anger. This has the advantage of letting people know right where they stand. But it produces "yes men" even among their most trusted subordinates. Subordinates will tend to distort the facts, on which sound decisions are so dependent, in order to escape the boss's anger.

So, we might conclude that there is nothing wrong with emotions. They are necessary and desirable. But let's recognize them for what they are and be careful how we let them dictate, or even influence our behavior.

WHERE ARE YOU GOING? WHY?

There is a question that I like to ask young people who face an important decision about their future: If you had Aladdin's lamp, and could have one wish granted when the genie emerges, where would you wish to be, and doing what, twenty years from now? It is interesting to watch their reaction. Some, of course, are too young to have thought that far ahead and should not be pressed for an immediate answer. Nevertheless, it starts them doing some serious thinking. Others know exactly what and where they'd like to be in twenty years, and again it is interesting to watch them set their course toward their goal.

It seems to me that no executives, even the younger sub-executives, are too young to answer this question for themselves. And the answer, if really honest, would give rise to other questions, which might help them detour around otherwise inevitable future frustrations, psychosomatic disabilities, and sometimes bitter disillusionment.

Given one wish which would be granted, where would you like to be, and doing what, twenty years from now? Have you good reasons for this wish? Write them down and look at them again and again. Do they hold up over a period of time? If so, is your present job leading toward this goal? If not, what changes in direction are you planning? To be sure, there will be many events occurring in the future which are beyond your control. But you'll be surprised at how much you can control your own destiny if you *know* where you want to go. On the other hand, you may be wishing for the moon. Unless you're training to be an astronaut, forget it and set a more realistic goal.

My old chief, Dr. Lee K. Frankel, from whom I learned so much, used to say: "Bill, don't waste your substance trying to rearrange the constellations of the universe. But watch them closely. There comes a time and place for everything. Be very sure you know what you wish to do, and that you know how to do it. Then when events have shaped themselves just right, move in, and move in fast."

This proved to be good counsel. It spared my energies. It increased my "frustration quotient," with which, as Alan Gregg used to say, every medical administrator must be generously endowed. One can manipulate events to a limited extent and there's no harm in trying, except the harm that one inflicts on himself by crying over spilled milk. More often than not, one must wait patiently for events to arrange themselves. But when they do, move in quick and with the assurance of a well worked out plan.

THE GOOD WITH THE BAD IN MOST JOBS

The question is, how do you *feel* toward your job? Few can answer this question "One hundred per cent O.K." Almost every job has components which are unpleasant, or at least parts that are less pleasant than others. If these are too numerous and too distasteful, you're in for a headache, either real or figurative. Is it worth it, or is it time to make a change that will lead more directly to your goal? It is the rare individual who before accepting a new job, or a promotion, can find and sample the skimmed milk that goes with the cream. Every job has its cream and it's on the top for all to see and sample. But what's underneath? It is said by the experts that milk is a universal food. That may be so, but I would add that too much milk can give you constipation.

If, on the other hand, you like the skimmed milk and find the cream delectable; if you really feel that this job is worthy of your mettle; if you find it interesting and challenging; if it is a pleasure to try your best to solve the riddles that come the way of every executive; if it is fun to use your ingenuity to overcome the obstacles in your race with competition—then you're doing all right, my friend. That forebrain will not bother you with too many tricks that you don't see through; it will help you, as only the subconscious can help, to be a smooth-functioning, well-co-ordinated, successful individual, well on his way to a goal which he thinks is worth attaining.

When I was in high school and already reading some of the medical books in my father's library, I commenced to develop some of the symptoms of whatever disease I was reading about, as was to be expected. (As I remember, spinal meningitis was one of the worst. It turned out to be a stiff back from cranking the old Ford on a certain cold morning.) My father would always listen gravely to my symptoms and examine me carefully. After this had gone on for some little time and he had finished the latest examination, he said: "Bill, you will always have aches and pains from time to time. We all do. If they persist, have them looked into just as I am doing for you now. They don't amount to anything ninety-nine times out of a hundred. Meantime, you have important work to do. You are an important person and, one day, you'll be a great doctor. You are far too important a person to be disabled by these minor aches and pains. As soon as you're sure you're all right, forget those minor symptoms and get that job done that you really didn't want to do."

This proved a good antidote for the neuroses which nearly all doctors have. So do most other people who amount to anything. One great psychiatrist says: "Thank God for the neuroses. Without them we'd all be inane and stupid." It's only when we don't recognize the neuroses for what they are that they may get us into trouble.

GOOD AND BAD PSYCHOLOGY

"Warning Signs of a Nervous Breakdown" was the headline on a recent popular magazine article. The writer had called me for advice on how to handle this assignment from his editor. My advice was simple: "Don't write it." He didn't, but instead came out with a fairly sensible article concerning our nervous tensions and what they can do to us. Nevertheless, his editor insisted on the scarehead on the cover. I have no doubt that the editor knew more about what it takes to sell a magazine than I. But it's bunk, nevertheless, and in my opinion did a public disservice. If a man is going to have a nervous breakdown, whatever that is, he had best not know it. If he's not going to have a nervous breakdown, this subject might scare him into it.

Among the best executives I have known are those who have a reasonable understanding of normal psychology, especially the mechanics, as we know them, of inter-personal relations. Among the worst executives I have known are those who have taken an ill-conceived course in abnormal psychology, too often disguised under the title of "Mental Health." There are a number of very good short courses for executives on mental health and a number of popular texts on those aspects of psychiatry which are most helpful to the executive. But deliver me from ever having to work for the executive who talks glibly of so-and-so being the "psychotic type," or that so-and-so is in one of his "periods of manic depressive psychosis—they're cyclic, you know," or that so-and-so is "in one of his manic phases and his advice should be disregarded until he calms down." A little knowledge is a dangerous thing in all of medicine, but especially in the field of psychiatry. This does not mean that the good executive should not know what medicine and psychiatry have to offer toward the solution of some of his problems. But he should also know what they do not have to offer.

One executive I knew became converted to "mental hygiene." He had finally "seen the light" and thought his company ought to have some of it. Not knowing a psychiatrist from a psychologist, he hired one who called himself, "an industrial social psychologist."

This man required furnishings and trappings for his tenth floor office such as had never been seen before in that factory. Among other requirements was a couch, which he insisted was necessary for his "analytical" work. This upset the purchasing department completely because there was a specific rule against couches in that place since the day one had been used there for purposes other than strictly business. Nevertheless, he got the couch with executive approval.

In due course, a supervisor referred to him an especially troublesome employee who had been on and off the job several times with recurrent "nervous breakdown." Little did he know, nor would he deign to find out, this man's record in the medical department, where he was known to be patently psychotic with occasional impulses toward suicide. Several times, while reclining on the couch, the employee threatened to jump out of the window. One day he did. The next day the industrial social psychologist was fired.

Now, this is not to condemn all social psychologists, even the "industrial" ones. Today they are much better trained than they were then and one of their first principles is to work as part of the medical team, where they are often very helpful. I cite this case simply to show that the executive had no knowledge of the limitations of the person he hired, nor did he take the trouble to seek advice from his medical director. Unwittingly, and with none but good intentions, he did not know the limitations of a psychologist, and unfortunately selected one who likewise did not know his own limitations. He might have been spared the trouble and expense over the couch had he known that the best trained clinical pyschologists today rarely, if ever, undertake psychoanalysis via the couch method except under close medical (*i.e.*, psychiatric) supervision. And finally, no psychologist or psychiatrist today will regard with anything but alarm even an idle threat of suicide, and will take every possible precaution to prevent it.

DEPRIVING MISFORTUNE OF ITS POWER

As stated at the beginning of this chapter, this is no place for a textbook on psychosomatic medicine or on psychiatry. Rather, the intention was to give the executive, who has been too busy becoming an executive to give much thought to his own mental and physical health, a little insight into what his unrecognized, and especially his subconscious, emotions may do to him as a result of that marvelous organ called the brain, and especially the forebrain, with its intricate system of circuits and, sometimes, short circuits. Lest what has been said here arouse undue apprehension, let me conclude the chapter by pointing out that the human personality is a marvelous and intricate thing. As an executive, yours is already superior to the average run of personalities. You have better health, both mental and physical, than most people. You work hard, but it is because you like to: and work *per se* never killed a normal individual.

As they do of all workers as well as the idle rich, the years will take their toll and your mental and physical mechanism will eventually run down. This inexorable process cannot be stopped. It can be retarded appreciably by taking good care of your physical mechanism, and by understanding to some extent at least some of the tricks of the forebrain, many of which you can circumvent. Some need help to do this. Your doctor will know whether you are one of these. You will have your ups and downs in business and at home. Good physical health and an ability to understand your own strengths and weaknesses will help you through the down periods and even give you added strength of character. As Seneca once said many years ago:

"Happy the man who can endure the highest and the lowest fortune. He who has endured such vicissitudes with equanimity, has deprived misfortune of its power."

CHAPTER 4

WORK, PLAY, AND TENSION: AVOIDING THE STRESS DISORDERS

LABORS OF CHILDHOOD

Did you ever watch young animals at play? I am told that all young animals play except camels, who seem to be born protesting this vale of tears and spend their whole lives in the same frame of mind. Thank goodness we don't face a population explosion of camels. There are already enough adult human beings who seem to spend their lives protesting. But even these confirmed "sour pusses" were once babies, and, chances are, they played and frolicked just like most young animals.

Relaxed and carefree as young animals seem to be, there is always a strenuous element in their play. It's how they learn to tense, strengthen and relax their young muscles and to co-ordinate the movements of their bones, tendons and muscles with their senses of smell, hearing, vision and balance. They are learning to become adults, strong, self-reliant and ready for self-preservation. But they have fun doing it! There seems to be no serious stress or strain, at least while they are young.

NOT CHILD LABOR

Did you ever watch the very young human infant first try to lift his head from the crib? As he awakes from a nap on his belly, there suddenly comes the urge to lift the head and see what's going on. Such effort usually requires a moment of grunting, straining and head-bobbing while the little face grows red with the effort. Then comes the good old bellow to notify the world that the nap is over. Just a few weeks later come his first efforts to turn over. This nearly always requires much grunting, straining and persistence, interspersed with moments of rest and usually some vocalization. Once over, with success achieved, the baby is obviously gratified. Now it's playtime; and arms, legs, head, eyes and voice are all in motion to the obvious pleasure of the infant and his parents. These are prodigious efforts of muscles, nerves and brain to do something that has to be done. Stress and strain, yes!—but it's all fun.

Next thing you know, he's up on the roof, or climbing a tree—more heroic efforts of muscles, brain and eye. But even though sometimes suffering cuts and bruises, he is easily comforted.

Children risk these hurts at least once because such adventures challenge young minds. They're fun and exciting. Stress and strain? Well, I should say so—both to clothing and body tissues, and, worst of all, to the heart and mind of parents. But it's all a part of the serious and pleasurable business of growing up—necessary, inevitable, compulsive. It's the only way children can develop their muscles, learn to co-ordinate, accumulate experiences to be stored in that growing forebrain and catalogued for future guidance.

WEAVING THE FABRIC OF CHARACTER

Many childhood experiences will be forgotten to the extent that they cannot be recalled to mind at will. But a behavior pattern is set up, and when this same mind and body, years later, finds itself in a situation similar to the one that resulted in youthful pain or pleasure, it will react the same way. That's why these early experiences, even as early as the cradle, are so important. Lifetime behavior patterns are being woven. The warp of the pattern might be called the hereditary genes contributed by the parents, and all their forebears. The woof of the pattern is all the complexities of the environment, many but not all of which can be controlled by the parents. The beauty and worth to the world of this new pattern depend largely on how successful the parents are in helping the child to make the best of his heredity (see Chapter 1), and so far as is humanly possible, to keep his childhood life-experiences in some kind of sensible, progressive balance.

THE LOOM OF THE GODS

One day when I was a school health director I was discussing child delinquency with the Superintendent of Schools and the Chief of Police of a little city renowned for its modern school system and its progressive police department. It was one of our regular monthly meetings to exchange information affecting our respective departments.

Said the school man, himself a leader in educational psychology: "Do you know, I think I could make almost anything I wanted to out of an average child, if from his birth through his tenth year I could have complete control of his successes and failures."

I said, "Now hold on, Professor, how about Joe Doaks' five-year-old? I just picked her up in the first grade with tuberculosis. You know that family, living in squalor down there by the old soap factory. This girl's illness could have been prevented. How would you go about that?"

"Yes, I know that family," said the Chief of Police. "They have nine children. Just last week we had to send the oldest boy to the reform school. This was his third major offense; his first was at age ten. How about him, Professor?"

"Now I said the *average* child," smiled the Professor, "and I'm not sure you heard that. However, I'll take you on, even with the Doaks children. Our school records show all six of the children now in school have normal intelligence, and they learn rapidly."

"Including the boy in the reform school?" asked the Chief.

"Yes, Chief. Actually, he's the brightest of all."

"Well!" snorted the Chief, "don't give me any more of those bright ones. That family has cost this city more money than any other five poor families in town; free hospital care every time there's another baby, on the relief rolls half the time, free visiting nurse visits, three jail sentences, and now the Doctor here will want this tuberculous child taken to the sanatorium for free care from the county."

"Yes," said the Professor, "too much failure and not enough success for poor Doaks and his whole family. That'll ruin anybody, especially a child." The Chief and I settled back for an interesting discussion.

"Suppose I *wanted* to make a child delinquent," said the Superintendent of Schools. "There's no better way to do it," he went on, "than to subject the child to one failure after another, beginning in infancy. His cries from discomfort, including hunger, are disregarded. He can find no way to attain success in relieving his discomfort. He fails again when he tries to obtain parental approval. He fails to get the love every baby needs. He grows up like a hungry little animal and soon learns to steal to gratify his needs. He fails to escape punishment, being cuffed about the home on every occasion. And when my truant officer finds him wandering the streets and not in school at age six, he is forced into school, another failure in his mind!

"It's a wonder my teachers can do anything with him, and they probably wouldn't try, except that his psychological tests indicate good learning capacity. With a superior teacher, one who studies his case, visits his family, works with the school nurse and the welfare workers, who sees that he goes to your school clinics, Doctor, and has his health improved, then we may possibly bring about his first mild success—a passing grade in school."

"But it's uphill work, Chief, and even our best efforts may be doomed to failure for us, and another failure for him. Some night, no one caring or knowing where he is, he runs into that little gang of teen-age boys you are now watching so closely, Chief. We know all of them, too, by the way, and are glad to work with you on their rehabilitation. But this night, they use his smallness and lack of scruples to crawl between the bars on the back window of that candy store and open the door for them. His share of the stolen goods may be one of the few successes in his bright, but mixed-up little mind. He gets a modicum of praise from the bigger boys—probably the first appreciation his poor starved little ego has ever had. So, he does it again. Sooner or later, your patrolman nabs him, Chief, and I must say that officer is one of your worthy disciples. Instead of taking him to his parents, where he would only get another beating, your juvenile department turned him over to the child welfare agency. But he's pretty far gone. Too much failure and not enough success."

Saddened by this story of cruelty and neglect, which I knew only too well, I said, "All right, Professor, a Divine Providence, we'll say, has given you full control of this poor kid's successes and failures, commencing at birth. How would you have handled him?"

"Well, it's not done by giving him all successes, either," said the Professor. "The extreme example of this is the so-called spoiled, pampered brat, getting anything he wants from his parents. He later becomes the arrogant, self-centered, selfish adolescent, demanding nothing but what he considers success and saying 'What I want, I want *now*!' He often gets it at any cost, a cost which may also bring him into the toils of the law."

"Yes," said the Chief, "we get that kind too, and I don't know which is worse."

"Success tempered with failure is the answer," said the Superintendent. "I would preferably alternate them fairly regularly. This is necessary to increase experience, strengthen character and develop the wisdom to live peacefully and constructively," said the Professor.

"The first successes should be little ones, and the first failures mild ones, gradually increasing the degree of each, and having each experience related to something the child did to account for each, and in which he understood just what he might have done differently to bring about the opposite result. There's a limit, of course, to the degree of failure I would have the heart to mete out to any child.

"We learn by doing, not by having things done to us. When we speak of teaching someone a lesson, we really mean giving the pupil an opportunity to learn. That's what the best teachers do, and what the best parents do. Some of the old guild masters were the most skilled at this. They gave the apprentice the things requiring the least skill first, then gradually the more difficult, expecting failures at the start, but always encouraging him to try again, until he developed great skills, his failures disappeared, and a new master was ready to train a new apprentice."

"But we're talking about a fanciful impossibility," said I. "No one could possibly control and alternate every success and failure in a child's life, let alone determine their degree."

"Of course," sighed the Professor, "we're just dreaming. But doesn't this make it a little easier for us to understand some of the reasons why one child is a delinquent and another makes a brilliant success of his life?"

"You're right!" said the Chief, "and I'm inclined to think that wise parents and teachers can do a great deal at least to modify the failures of the child who has already had too many, and to guide him toward a few more successes for a while."

"Chief," exclaimed the Professor, "for a policeman, you're the best educational psychologist I ever saw!"

"Professor, I envy that compliment to the Chief," said I. "Could I qualify too, if I added that life is often rugged, if not cruel, to some people, through no fault of their own, and that when the family is struck by such a disaster as death or prolonged illness, wise parents and teachers can often soften the blow for the child by giving him increased attention and help for a while."

"You both qualify for an honorary degree," laughed the Superintendent of Schools. "When we meet next month I expect to learn enough from each of you to earn a police chief's badge and an honorary M.D."

THE SHUTTLE BETWEEN WORK AND PLAY

So life, from the moment of birth, is a series of experiences, some gratifying, many unpleasant. But whatever those little unfocused eyes in the cradle may live to see, that baby will start within the first few weeks to strive. Even without attention from parents or nurse, he begins to get ready for adulthood. And he really works at it grunting, pulling, pushing, kicking, finally creeping, then walking and climbing and ball playing. Much of it is playing; it's fun—but it's work too.

Then, where does stress, strain and tension come in? At what age do we commence to avoid work, and why? Why do strain and stress seem fun to the child, yet are considered by some to be harmful to adults? Are they really harmful? Can it be that stress becomes harmful only when it involves some unpleasantness? If so, how about that time you fell out of the apple tree and broke your leg? Unpleasant, wasn't it, but didn't you try it again and do it successfully?

Would you, a successful executive, really enjoy a life completely free of tension, frustration, worry? Would you really want every effort you make crowned with success—no failures? Let us study these questions a few moments.

THE TOUGH THREAD OF STRESS

First, what is stress? Well, it derives from the Latin "strictus," which means "to bind tight; to subject to the action of external forces, especially overstrain." To engineers the limits of stress are the "breakpoint," that is, the point where the action of external forces causes the material to fracture or disintegrate. We shall see later that the human organism also has its "breakpoint." But long before the breakpoint comes for humans, certain demonstrable changes take place in the body mechanism when they are subjected to continuous stress or overstrain.

If we follow the work of Hans Selye and others, we see that human stresses arise from emotions, many of them rather primitive and many of them unrecognized except by the subconscious mind. Among these more primitive emotions are fear or fright which automatically prepares the body for "flight or fight." Survival often depended upon the effectiveness of this preparation. Pursued by an enemy, both animal and man exerted prodigious effort either to run away, climb a tree or otherwise escape. Lacking an opportunity to escape, they faced the enemy for a fight.

In either case the adrenal glands, lying above but not directly connected with the kidneys, and secreting a number of hormones, among then adrenin, go into immediate action. They pour extra adrenin into the blood stream, which working with the other glands producing other hormones, prepares the body for the emergency. The blood supply to the stomach and intestines is markedly reduced, that to the heart and other muscles markedly increased; the heart beats faster, blood pressure rises, and breathing is quickened. This comes about through a neuro-chemical reaction which constricts the blood vessels to the parts of the body not needed in the emergency, and dilates the vessels to the parts needed for flight or fight. It is an interesting mechanism, not yet fully understood, but we do know it is triggered by the brain, which in turn is activated by sight, sound, smell or the other special senses. And we do know that the adrenin increase in the blood can be measured with some accuracy. We also know what adrenin does to the body by experimental work with animals and even human volunteers. The adrenals have a powerful effect on the body. They often save it. They may destroy it.

We often observe that soldiers in combat or other human beings in peril exert "superhuman efforts." They perform feats they would never attempt in the absence of this preparation. They are often as much astonished by such feats as is their enemy. When badly frightened we lose our appetite and cannot eat. Often when the danger is over, but never *during* the superhuman effort, the frightened one is nauseated or actually vomits the food which could not be digested because of decreased blood supply and other temporary arrests in the digestive process. Not infrequently bladder and bowels become involuntary. After it's over, he may get the "shakes" as though he had a chill. These symptoms are all due to the excess adrenin. We can reproduce them in unfrightened human beings by injecting adrenin under the skin. The antidote for excess adrenin is exercise, to taper off the stimulation left over in the muscles. Thats why we pace the floor when our wife is having a baby. We're scared and can't do anything about it. That's why golf, or a brisk walk, or a swim is good for us when we're afraid, worried or frustrated—as we shall see.

Well, these are among the actual physical changes which take place as a result of stress arising from emotions, primitive though such emotions may be. They are by no means under our conscious control. They are automatic and have often accounted for survival of the human race in times of danger and stress.

TO DESTROY OR PRESERVE?

Strangely enough, many of the less primitive emotions and feelings—such things as worry, anxiety, frustration and mental fatigue—will automatically set this same mechanism in motion. We often worry because, even though unconsciously, we fear something. We're afraid that we can't do this job right; we're afraid that we can't earn enough to pay our bills; having done something our conscience tells us is wrong, we are afraid someone will find out about it. We're afraid that we're about to have a nervous breakdown, or that a loved one will not recover from an illness, or that we won't get that promotion.

FEAR, WORRY, FRUSTRATION

Worry is a tricky thing. Like anxiety, it frequently becomes a habit which is hard to break, but unless it becomes excessive, irrational and habitual, a little worry is good for us.

One wise doctor of my acquaintance, listening repeatedly to the endless string of worries which were upsetting his patient, decided that they were all really minor and that as soon as one was dissipated the patient would find another. The patient had the worry habit. He finally advised: "Now I'll tell you what you do. Listen carefully to me. At a certain time every day you take a half hour out by yourself when no one will distract your mind. Then you sit down and worry. Just worry. Think of all the things that worry you. Don't do anything else. At the end of thirty minutes, stop worrying and get busy. If worries come into your mind during the rest of the day don't bother with them then. Make a note of them and worry about them at the appointed time tomorrow." In due time the patient commenced to forget what it was she was going to worry about at the appointed hour. Then she worried because she had nothing to worry about. At this point she convinced herself, as no other person could have convinced her, that most of her worries were foolish.

Anxiety is closely akin to worry, often necessary and beneficial, as we shall see. But it, too, often becomes a habit, a state of mind, and it can grow into an unbearable burden. The psychiatrists identify what they call a "chronic anxiety state," a form of mental illness which is difficult to treat, but I am by no means convinced that the individual oppressed by many anxieties develops any such mental illness. More likely, the mental illness was there anyway and happened to take this form.

Frustration and mental fatigue are in the same category as worry and fear, producing the same stress phenomena in the body, except that the individual is more often the victim of circumstances which seem beyond his control, rather than suffering from a habit pattern of unwarranted worry and fear.

The point I want to make here is that these less primitive emotions, according to Selye and others, automatically and without our knowing it, set up that wonderful old defense mechanism, which preserved our lives and that of our forebears. In modern civilization we may be afraid of this or that, but we can't climb a tree or run away; we can't enter into physical combat with a boss who won't promote us or who gives us too big a job to do. Yet, here is this same old mechanism working. And there is no doubt that it was revived and enhanced by our childhood experiences. They weren't all fun, like the time that big bully beat up on us, or we fell through the ice and nearly drowned. Due to the inevitable worry, anger, fear, frustration and fatigue of modern life, that old mechanism is pouring too much adrenin into our blood stream too frequently; our heart beats faster than it should; our blood pressure rises; we feel short of breath; our digestive system is upset. But we can't work it off by fight or flight.

Selye and others go on to show that this automatic defense mechanism will in time actually narrow and harden the arteries, producing the same pathological tissue changes we saw in the caged monkey and the monkey with the electrode in his brain.

According to the best authorities today, high blood pressure, hardening of the arteries, coronary disease, apoplexy and certain forms of kidney disease are caused by a number of things, including infectious diseases, faulty diet, overweight, inadequate exercise. But they may also be caused by long continued emotional disturbances such as those we have been discussing.

HOW TOUGH IS STRESS?

So that's where stress comes in. "Binding tight" by the "action of external forces" which, if continued long enough, will bring us to the "breakpoint." Of course, the breakpoint in humans does not necessarily mean "fracture or disintegration." It may simply mean that we are growing mature enough to throw off the parental yoke, which some never do. It may mean finally deciding that we're on the wrong track with the present job, so we throw it over and find another. It may mean having a showdown with the board of directors so that we and they know just where we stand henceforth.

It is the wise executive who can discern the major issues on which he must take a firm stand and can prepare himself for the breakpoint. When he does this, the "stress effect" is no more serious than the foot race or the football game he won or lost at college. So far as our physiology is concerned, it makes little difference whether we win or lose. The strain is over. Fear, anger, worry and frustration subside. The adrenals return to normal activity; high blood pressure and rapid pulse disappear; the stomach and intestines get their normal blood supply and the digestive juices flow again. The possibility of permanent injury from stress only occurs when it is continuous over a long period, and the individual feels he can do nothing about it.

From the psychological standpoint, losing a decisive contest may harm certain people. These are the individuals who feel they must *always* win. They are the ones who must have what they want and have it now. Rather immature, isn't it? The extremes of difference between these two types of executives are illustrated by those who committed suicide during the depression of the early 1930's, and those who, though equally ruined financially, staged a courageous and successful comeback.

But, you may say, how about the stresses of childhood which were referred to as fun? It's not easy to learn to walk and finally to run fast enough to win a race. That's strain and stress, as I have said. But childhood stress is for the most part voluntary; hence there is considerably less conflict between what the child wants to do and what someone makes him do. To be sure, there is some frustration, especially when the teen-ager is not allowed to drive the car, or the eight-year-old has to wash his face and hands before dinner, when he is *so* hungry. But these are minor frustrations and temporary. If they cause high blood pressure, and they seldom do in children, it is soon relieved.

What it comes down to, then, is that stress and strain, hard work and tension are all good for us, whether we like them or not. Without them we could not learn to walk, win contests, solve problems, make a better mousetrap, beat our competitors. It's the fellow who doesn't try who gets nowhere. The one who tries, even though he fails, is the one who will try again, and with even greater effort and with more skill because of his previous experience. Even though he doesn't win the complete success he expected, he is better off with half a loaf than none, and he'll do better next time, if he has any wit at all. Success, on the other hand, especially by dint of hard work, hard striving, careful planning, and determined effort, tends to engender success. It makes the next contest easier.

On the other hand, it cannot be denied that stress is often harmful. Why? Well, the answer is simple: too much of it. It is all a matter of balance. Left to their own devices the infant and the young animal will struggle and strain at play until something tells them they are tired. And here, I sometimes think, they are wiser than we are. When tired, they rest. Nature's balance of work and rest is well observed by them. Among adults, however, the runner in the mile race can't quit and rest because he's tired at the half mile. Nor can the business executive quit and rest because he's tired before the end of a strenuous session at the bargaining table.

Like the miler, he has to see it through, win or lose. But the miler doesn't get up immediately and run another mile. Yet that's just what many executives try to do. "I don't have time to be tired," they say. Well, sooner or later they will and meanwhile they will gradually develop some of the stress disorders, including mental fatigue.

MENTAL FATIGUE

Mental fatigue is one of the hardest things to recognize in one's self, unless one is on the lookout for it. But your subordinates recognize it in you. Quite unconsciously you become short tempered, you snap at them, the faults which they all have seem worse than usual and you lose patience with them. The same goes with your wife and family. The younger children may leave the dinner table crying over some words of yours. The older ones whisper to Mama, "What's the matter with Daddy?" They all seem noisier and more quarrelsome than usual.

It's your fault, Bud! You brought it about because you're mentally fatigued. Take a deep breath and look at yourself in the mirror. A little grayer than usual, aren't you? Mouth sags at the corners, doesn't it? Aren't those vertical wrinkles in your forehead deeper than they used to be, and don't they make you look crankier or more worried?

Yes, you've got it my friend—mental fatigue, and you'd better do something about it now. If you'll go to your doctor, he'll weigh its seriousness and discuss sensible plans for its relief. If a critical situation in your business will not permit immediate slowdown, he'll help tide you over. Meanwhile, he'll be on the lookout for the even more serious danger signs: mounting blood pressure, dyspepsia, constipation or diarrhea and maybe ulcer. He may insist that you shift gears and slow down as soon as possible, or ask how soon you can take a vacation.

The man with executivitis will disagree, but in my view the one characteristic which marks a good executive is equanimity. He above all others must keep a cool head, especially in times of stress. He is there to back up the line and call the signals. He can do this only by setting himself a pace that will avoid mental fatigue and the concomitant stress disorders. With appropriate delegation of authority to competent subordinates he can do this, and plan a little time off to maintain or regain his equanimity. When he "blows up," as he obviously does when he gets short-tempered, the whole place blows up too.

I once had a patient who was a minister. No one I ever knew practiced the golden rule as fully as he did. He was kindly, understanding, beloved equally by the saints and the sinners in his parish, with a happy combination of goodness, gentleness and forcefulness in his philosophy of life which inspired his sermons. I was looking for him one day to comfort a patient, one of his flock who was going to die. But he was nowhere to be found. His wife explained that he often took a half day or even a day or two off, and that no one knew where he was during these periods, but he always told her when he would be back. (He did return in ample time to comfort the departing one.) Later I asked, "Tell me, where do you go when you disappear occasionally?" He quickly replied: "Doctor, at times the troubles of my parishioners are so great that I have to have time off all by myself just to meditate." I often wish that some of my friends who are really great executives would take more time off, "just to meditate."

BALANCE AND PACE

So now we come to the purpose of this chapter. Too much stress over too long a period of time can destroy you. Little or no stress, and you're little better than a vegetable, accomplishing nothing throughout life but your own comfort. It is all a matter of balance between stress and relaxation, between work and play, between setting yourself too stiff a pace or one which your own particular physical and mental endowments will stand as long as you want them to.

Fortunately, we can, if we will, learn to gauge our own strengths and weaknesses. Some of the strengths we can develop into even greater strengths. Some of the weaknesses we can overcome or circumvent if we recognize them and are willing to try hard enough. But in the main, the man born with the build of a bulldog will never change his build to that of a greyhound. To try to make one into the other is impossible. Fortunately, too, in the absence of undue influence by parents or others, we tend to seek the kind of work we like to do, and that's usually what we are best at. Liking it, we become better and better at it, so that really nature is helping us set our balance, just as she does with young animals. So most of us get along all right, in the main.

EXECUTIVES' PREROGATIVES

Some people get their best work done when they work at a steady pace, so many hours a day, so many weeks a year. This is a questionable practice for an executive whose pressures vary with the exigencies of the business and who must be ready for the many critical situations arising throughout the year.

Punching the Time Clock

Generally speaking, the executive cannot be a time clock puncher. Special privilege goes with special responsibility and the one who denies this was really not cut out to be a good executive. There will be times when he must work early and late, but there should be other times when he can come in late in the morning and leave early enough for a round of golf before dinner. This is all to the good. With the executive, it's results that count and a steady pace of forty hours a week may not always be the best way to get the best results. Emergencies cannot always be taken care of in the eight-hour day, so he puts in twelve or even sixteen hours. That's all right for a while, but it could become a habit. Very few men can keep up such a pace for long.

The young wags on Wall Street, looking forward to the time when their fortunes equal the bosses' say boastfully: "Watch me twenty years from now. If I have to show up in my office any time between Memorial Day and Labor Day, I'll think that I've not yet arrived."

An interesting example of the time clock failing to measure accomplishment occurred recently when government auditors assayed to apply the usual man-hour measurements to the research grants awarded the scientists of a certain medical school. Dividing the total allocation for salaries by the assumed man-hours devoted to the job, they reported that the salaries far exceeded those customary in Washington.

Replied the dean of that medical school: "This conclusion is based upon a faulty premise, namely, that my scientists work the same number of hours per week as are required of civil service employees. They do not. I have made a time study of the actual hours devoted to this research project by the responsible investigator and his staff. During critical experiments they frequently work around the clock, resuming their teaching and other duties next morning with little or no sleep for a day or two. At least half of this staff works throughout the weekend. Counting study time at home and in the libraries, a paper-sack lunch eaten between manipulations in the laboratory, and no time out for the usual Washington coffee-break, my figures show that these men receive less than half the civil service scale in Washington."

Like the executive, the scientist's work is never done. No one can measure the hours of thought devoted to current problems by scientist and executive in the still of night, during a golf game or even during a game of bridge. What started Isaac Newton thinking about the laws of gravitation? If the legend is true, he was sitting under an apple tree when the apple dropped. Working? No, meditating. And out of his meditations came the formulation of the laws of gravitation and the wonderful new mathematical system called calculus.

Yes, the true executive is a man apart. He is different from other men, most of whom *must* punch the time clock if we are to have any systematic rate of production anywhere. I stress this point because in the interests of his physical and mental health, the executive *must* be free to set his own pace.

The Relaxed Type

Some executives work best when well relaxed. This is not laziness. It's an indication that they know best their own strengths and limitations. If pushed to the point of prolonged tension, they blow up in one way or another. They actually become sick, as any medical director in a large establishment will tell you. These are the men who should be freed from the time clock entirely; they should have frequent days off without criticism, so long as their results are satisfactory. And they should have two vacations a year of two to four weeks each. After all, what's so sacred about this vacation business as far as executives are concerned? This particular type of man will wear longer and produce more good results for more years if you see to it that he remains relaxed.

One medical director of a large industry was confronted with a problem, the solution of which illustrates the needs of this particular type of executive. The man was an expert in a highly technical field. He was a near-genius, no doubt about it. But since coming to the plant his illness-absence record was the cause of much concern. He had been out sick nearly a third of the working days during the past year. No question about his illnesses. They were genuine. The question was, can this man stand the gaff in this business, or should we get rid of him?

After studying the man's responsibilities and the ingenious way in which he met them, according to his fellows and his immediate superiors, it was evident to the medical director that no one else could do this tricky job so well. But he was being pushed too hard by the traditional time clock complex. The doctor therefore recommended that the man work only four days a week and that he be ordered to take three weeks vacation in summer and three weeks in the winter. Fortunately, the president of the concern was willing to see the man himself and make this schedule obligatory, and to say that he would defend it if any questions were raised. His illnesses stopped completely and he got more done, more skillfully on this short working schedule than others did on forty hours a week with annual vacations of two weeks.

Getting Steam Up

There are other good executives who work best only after "getting up a head of steam." They need time to fire up their boilers. Once steam is up, they tear into their work with tremendous energy, on and on into the night, to the great distress of their secretarial staff. Whoever had a more overwhelming executive job than Winston Churchill? If I understand his biographers correctly, he was this kind of man. According to Emil Ludwig, Bismarck was another. He rose at a late hour, breakfasted in his chamber in a leisurely manner, seeing no one on business. Then he rode his horse for an hour or two and had luncheon. Finally about midafternoon, steam was up, and his office became a veritable beehive of activity, working far into the night and getting enormous amounts done and done well. Ludwig makes the point that people are born to be early risers and early retirers, or to be late risers and late retirers and they do their best work if this diurnal or nocturnal rhythm is not disturbed. They are the devil to work with, to be sure, but there are some top executive jobs filled by such people. They, too, are setting their own pace.

THE INEVITABILITY OF TENSION

To summarize this chapter, we find that tension, stress and strain are inevitable for any executive worth his salt. On the whole, and for the healthy person they are beneficial throughout life, commencing in infancy. They enable us to grow up, to gain strength, experience and wisdom, to win contests, arise to greater achievement, and add to the world's progress. They can be, and often are harmful, however, when too long continued, and when not interspersed with periods of relaxation such as that imposed by nature on the very young.

To strike a proper balance between work and play is especially important for the executive in the interests of his health. In the ordinary exigencies of big business many things may happen to upset that balance. Whether the executive will regain it or will fall depends on his recognizing these exigencies, comparing them with his own limitations and making provision for them in setting his pace. He needs considerable leeway in attaining the balance best suited to him, and in setting his pace. If the job requirements are such as to throw him off balance repeatedly, or to demand a pace of which he is not capable, then he must give serious thought to whether he is in the job for which he is best suited. He must choose between his job and his health. Too often, the decision is made in favor of the job, and health is irretrievably lost.

CHAPTER 5

WHAT MAKES US TICK—FOODS AND NUTRITION

"WHAT You Eat Today Will Walk and Talk Tomorrow"

This macabre sign in the window of a so-called "natural foods" store did not exactly enhance my appetite. A bit gruesome, isn't it? You look at your ham sandwich and wonder if that slice of pork will grunt and squeal tomorrow. Will it walk on four legs, or will I? Or is this really the transmigration of souls wherein this little pig went to market and learned to walk and talk and become part of a human?—And this delectable asparagus, 50¢ a pound it is, at the first of the season; or $1.65 for a plate of five flavorsome stalks with hollandaise at the Waldorf. Does it become part of me, or am I to be a part of it? Will my bones and juices eventually help fertilize its offspring many generations hence by being washed down into that fertile delta of the San Joaquin River where asparagus grows so lush? I once knew a good Chinese gardener who collected dead cats. Said there was nothing better to assure the successful transplantation of a young cherry tree.

Many years ago, in San Francisco, it became necessary to move and vacate the old Masonic Cemetery to make room for new houses. It had been filled to capacity and unused for two generations, and city ordinances now prohibited the establishment of new cemeteries within the city limits. I remember how Dr. William C. Hassler, the long-time great health officer of the City and

County, fumed because his bureau of vital statistics was able to locate the relatives of these dead in only about one out of twenty cases. Nevertheless, they were moved with due solemnity and the markers restored in the new location. Those old, long forgotten bones must have leached into the soil well, for the people living there now are said to have the finest gardens in the City.

"Well," you may say justifiably, "what a way to start to talk about foods and nutrition." " 'Twan't me, honest," I say. Blame the natural foods store. They got me thinking along this line. And do you know, I believe there's food for thought, if not for the appetite, in "what you eat today, walks and talks tomorrow."

Anyway, when we come to think about what makes us tick, foods and nutrition are a good place to start, since eating is an increasing pleasure for some and an increasing problem for others as we grow older. Almost everyone today is talking about diets for this and that, mainly to control or find excuses for being overweight. Many of them know as little about diets as the little girl who was sent to the druggist and said,

"My mother has stomach trouble and wants to diet."

The puzzled druggist said, "Very well, what kind would you like?"

Said the little girl, "She didn't say, but if she's got to dye it, I like red best."

NUTRITION RESEARCH

The science of nutrition in the past fifty years has undergone development almost as amazing as that of nuclear physics. Vast areas of research have opened up and are being pursued on many fronts by the Department of Agriculture, the National Health Institutes, the National Nutrition Foundation, and by many universities. So maybe some of the things we learned about foods in college hygiene are no longer true.

The exact physio-chemical mechanism by which foods are transformed into living tissues in the body is still largely a mystery. Yet, of course, it happens every day we live. As pointed out by Heller in his classic little book *Of Mice, Men and Molecules* (New

York: Charles Scribner's Sons, 1960), we still know very little about the molecular physics of any living organism. We have come a long way in nutrition research, but we have a still longer way to go.

WHAT ABOUT VITAMINS?

Many millions of dollars are spent by the public today in buying vitamins of assorted colors, kinds and composition to feed the family as a supplement to their regular diet. "Vitamin specials" are frequently advertised in drug and grocery stores. "Dietetic food" stores do a brisk business in selling cut-rate vitamins in various combinations as pills, liquids or creams to rub on the skin. Many of these products (I was about to say most) are worthless and the great majority of people who buy them don't need them. A few do. Some interesting things about vitamins are these:

First, they are necessary to life and health, and the complete lack of them or even the continued, marked reduction of any one of them can cause illness.

Exploration of the globe or sea was greatly hampered for centuries by whole crews being disabled or dying of scurvy. Finally, the British "limeys" showed how to escape it by provisioning their ships with lime juice and other fresh fruits and vegetables. They did not know that Vitamin C prevents scurvy or that it was found in fresh fruits and vegetables. But this discovery contributed greatly to Britain's superiority on the sea.

Many oriental population groups subsisting largely on polished rice suffer high death and disability rates because of beri-beri due to lack of one of the "B" group of vitamins—thrown away with the husks when the rice is "refined."

Indeed, it is only rather recently that the dread black-tongue-fever, or pellagra, has come under control, in some of the rural counties of our own South by correcting vitamin deficiencies in the diet—too much corn pone and sow belly and not enough red meats and fresh vegetables.

Before the World War II, I helped entertain some very able Japanese nutritionists who were concerned over the lack of Vitamin B in the national diet of Japan. They had concluded that the cheapest way to remedy this was to encourage the eating of the plentiful grasshoppers, and they assured me that they were quite palatable when properly prepared. Africans, apparently, know this. Some tribes customarily serve deep-fat-fried grasshoppers as one of their feast delicacies. One wonders how often new articles of food have been accepted over the centuries because of a craving for certain vitamins which were lacking in the diet and plentiful in the new article. Who, for instance, had the courage to eat the first snail, or oyster, or the "love-apple" tomato for that matter, which has become second only to the citrus fruits as a source of Vitamin C.

Some who have been observing people as long as I have will remember the frequency with which we used to see bowlegged folks. It was said they had learned to walk before their bones could bear the weight. That was true, but what made their bones so soft? They had had rickets in infancy. Their mothers had not yet learned how to make them like cod-liver oil. Today we rarely see a really bowlegged person. The Vitamin D in fish oils together with sunshine for the infant prevents it.

So there's no doubt that vitamins, all that we know of now, and probably some we have yet to discover, are necessary to good health.

The second peculiar thing about vitamins is that they come in very small amounts. You might say that only a whiff is necessary to keep you well.

A third peculiarity, not entirely limited to vitamins, is that they are perishable. Wilting, the spraying of water on vegetables on the market stands, unrefrigerated storage and drying, destroy or greatly reduce the natural vitamins in our foods, especially those soluble in water such as Vitamin C. Milling and refining of grains, including rice, removes most of the vitamins. Perhaps the commonest cause of reducing both needed vitamins and minerals is improper cooking. Vegetables soaked in water before cooking and boiled a long time have few vitamins left. And the minerals go down the sink when the water is drained off. The virtues of waterless and pressure cookery as well as low-heat roasting of meats are well presented by Adele Davis in her *Let's Cook It Right* (New York: Harcourt Brace & Co., 1947). Many men of my acquaintance have found this little book good reading.

Fortunately, considering the increasing distance between food producer and urban markets, refrigeration, canning and quick freezing preserve most, though not all, the vitamin content of food. But the family who can eat vegetables and fruits the same day they're picked is still most fortunate.

The fourth peculiarity of vitamins is that, whatever infinitesimal amounts are present in the food we eat, those amounts will be seized and used by the body. Any excess vitamins in foods, or in the pills we take are, with the exceptions of Vitamins A and D cast off through the kidneys or bowels. They are not stored for a rainy day.

My grandfather never tired of telling the story of the time he was called to attend my great uncle, who regarded all doctors with much suspicion, but allowed as how he felt pretty terrible this time and thought it might be safe to trust this one medical member of the family. True to the homeopathic tradition of that day, Grandfather asked him many detailed questions as to just where he hurt and what kind of hurt was it, what made it hurt worse and what made it better. Then he called for two half glasses of water with a separate teaspoon for each, put a few drops of pulsatilla diluted one part to ten million in one glass, stirred it carefully and gave the patient exactly one teaspoonful. Then he put a few drops of aconite, similarly diluted, in the other glass and stirred it carefully. After ten minutes, feeling the patient's pulse and counting his respirations the while, he gave him one teaspoonful from that glass. By that time, Uncle Peacey was feeling better. Grandfather left careful instructions for him to take a spoonful from one glass, then from the other every half hour until he went to sleep, and said that he would be back in the morning to see how he was and to replenish his medicine.

Just as Grandfather was retiring for the night, Auntie Peacey came running over, there being no telephone, and gasped,

"Come quick, Doctor! William has drunk all of both those glasses of medicine and he's unconscious!"

Grandfather, not too concerned, patiently put on his trousers again and his stiff white shirt with the ruby stud in it, plus the detachable cuffs that he always wore except when delivering a baby, and with his frock coat tails blowing behind him, walked over to Uncle Peacey's again. He found him sound asleep, not unconscious, and not wishing to be disturbed. When he was finally awake, Grandfather said,

"Will, I told you to take only one teaspoonful of each of those medicines, alternating every half hour until you went to sleep. That was only an hour ago, and here the medicine is all gone!"

"Sure, Doctor," replied my Great Uncle. "I've always believed that if a little bit of something was good for a fellow, a whole lot of it must be better."

The moral of the story was what Grandfather loved best. He would always conclude by saying,

"Suppose I had been an allopath (regular doctor) instead of a homeopath, and had left him some Fowler's solution (arsenic) or strychnine to be taken in small doses. He'd have died of rat poisoning that very night."

The moral of this story with respect to vitamins is that you don't need much. It's not true that if a little is good, a lot is better. Your body can't use but a tiny bit, your miraculously selective digestive absorption will find that little micromilligram of vitamin that nature put in your food and put it to good use for you. And if you poke more than a tiny bit into your gullet, it goes right through you and does nobody any good but the seller.

WHEN SUPPLEMENTS ARE NEEDED

Now this is not to say that no one needs supplementary vitamins. Generally speaking, a normal well-balanced diet will contain all you need of all the vitamins we know and some we don't know. However, there are some people who for reasons prescribed by the doctor are denied a completely balanced diet. Perhaps the commonest are those who must cut down calories in order to reduce excessive weight. Another group are those who must forego certain foods because of allergies or some damage in the digestive tract. Then, too, there are some people who apparently neither absorb certain vitamins as they should, nor synthesize their own vitamins as they should. Some upset their vitamin balance with too much alcohol. Finally, there are said to be a few who, though not obviously suffering from a vitamin deficiency, have what some doctors call "preclinical" signs of a deficiency such as may follow a serious illness or extensive surgery. And some women may need added amounts of certain vitamins and minerals during pregnancy.

These people need supplementary vitamins of one kind or another (seldom all). But they should be prescribed by a doctor, given only so long as needed in just the dosage needed. And finally, as with all drugs of any kind, "the best is none too good." The extra cost of patronizing a reputable druggist who handles reputable products of known potency and purity, is well worth it.

Avitaminosis, or actual illness caused by lack of vitamins, is indeed a rare occurrence in this country. It is almost unknown among medium- and high-income families. The once exception is rickets in infancy. Nearly all babies need the Vitamin D in fish-liver oils. Otherwise, the adequate and abundant diet of the great majority of American families makes it hard to understand the enormous sale of bottled vitamins.

BASIC FOOD ELEMENTS AND CALORIES

A quick glance at the chart of the basic food elements distributed by the U. S. Department of Agriculture will renew our knowledge of the fundamentals of a well-balanced diet. This chart, or something like it, such as those prepared by the Metropolitan Life Insurance Company and various university departments of home economics, should be readily accessible in every home kitchen across the land. It should be familiar not only to the homemaker but the whole family, especially Papa.

The adult members of the family, including teen-agers when

they are overweight, should have a pretty clear general idea of caloric values of the commonest classes of foods. Calorie charts are available in booklets, wheels and notebooks in most stationery stores and should be generally understood.

THE BUSINESSMAN'S LUNCH

The dietary habits of some otherwise intelligent businessmen often astound me—especially the businessman's lunch.

I can understand a man being hungry. There's something wrong with him if he isn't hungry at appropriate intervals. And even if he's engaged in the laudable enterprise of controlling his weight, I can understand his succumbing to temptation now and then, especially under the attraction of one of his favorite dishes, or the stimulation of a Rotary Club or Chamber of Commerce luncheon meeting, or even more especially when the little woman isn't there to keep tab on his intake.

But when a man drinks a glass of Metrecal at his desk to reduce his weight and then goes on to eat a full luncheon every day in the week, it beats me. Or when a man says he'll have a light luncheon today, "Have to watch the calories, you know!" and then eats half a dozen ripe olives, a buttered roll, cream soup, spaghetti with meat sauce, cheese cake with well creamed and sweetened coffee, feeling noble because he passed up the oysters, steak, baked potato, lettuce and tomato salad and baked apple, which he would have preferred, I wonder what he's got to feel noble about. Certainly not his ability to add up calories, nor his conception of a well-balanced diet. More about weight control later.

But now we're still talking about the fundamentals of nutrition and a well-balanced diet in order to get all the food elements we need as well as those necessary vitamins without buying them at a drug store.

PROTEINS

Proteins are called the building blocks of the body. Found largely in meats, including fish and fowl, in milk, cheese and eggs and some grains and vegetables, they are especially needed by the young for growth and by the adult for repair of body tissues which are constantly wearing out. They have fewer calories per gram than do carbohydrates or fats. Hence our friend would have done much better calorie-wise to have had the steak he preferred (especially if it were broiled) than to have chosen the high-calorie carbohydrate spaghetti and the high-calorie little-meat-and-much-fat meat sauce. Protein in adequate amounts is essential throughout life. Actually, many adults, and especially those with limited means who are aging, do not get their full daily requirement of protein. Protein, *per se,* especially if relatively free of fats, need not be greatly limited in a weight-reducing diet.

CARBOHYDRATES

Carbohydrates have been called the fuel for the body's fires, and believe it or not, you are burning fuel to produce energy every second so long as you're alive. The carbohydrates are the starches and sugars. They have higher caloric values per unit of weight than the proteins, but not as much as the fats. They are a source of quick energy and a very necessary part of the normal diet. Even diabetics who must avoid certain types and amounts of sugars are usually allowed some starchy foods. Carbohydrates form a high percentage of the bulk of all sweets and of breads, biscuits, pastries, and the "pastas" like noodles, spaghetti and ravioli.

When you add shortening to flour, then cook it with sweets for cake or pie, then top it with syrup or cream, you're not concerned with reducing the number of calories you eat that day. But how good these dishes are! When you serve spaghetti with butter or fatty meat sauce and you are concerned about your overweight, better skip a rich sweet dessert that meal. Yet, how good these farinaceous dishes really are, be they of Italian, French, Spanish or Chinese origin.

CUMULATIVE CALORIES

Sad to say, calories, unlike vitamins, do accumulate in the form of body fat. But, if you're watching your weight, you need not necessarily be denied these tasty carbohydrate dishes. Just make a mental note of it and next day see if you can't be satisfied with a fresh fruit and cottage cheese salad for lunch, the cottage cheese made from skimmed milk, of course, and if salad dressing is a must, one made with very little oil.

That's one comfort about dieting for overweight. It isn't like swearing off smoking or drinking. You don't have to take a pledge against anything. If you feel like a nice dish of ham hocks and sauerkraut, with a tankard of ale, go ahead and have them. But try to make up for the "binge" by cutting down the next few days.

THE SWEET TOOTH ACHE

A word more about sugars. Some people claim to have a "sweet tooth." They don't feel satisfied until they've had something sweet with or between meals. I can sympathize with this craving for I used to think I had a sweet tooth myself. But for years, now, in the interests of controlling my weight, I have not eaten desserts regularly. I find that saccharine, which has no calories and is a harmless chemical, seems to pacify my sweet tooth when used in the coffee. Saccharine or Sucaryl may also be used instead of sugar to sweeten desserts.

The natural, simple sugars of ripe fruits are easily digestible. Some believe that the taste for refined table sugar is an acquired taste. But what a hold it gets on the young, growing child especially. They just can't seem to get enough candy and sweetened drinks. Well, maybe they need the energy it gives them and perhaps it does no harm, especially if taken after meals, followed by a tooth brushing.

The bacteria between the teeth do seem to thrive on sugars, producing an acid which harms the tooth enamel and causes cavities. This danger is reduced by prompt tooth brushing, or even rinsing the mouth with water, each time after eating candy. I have known many children who have rarely, if ever, tasted candy and seem to have no craving for it. They have been given ample diets, including lots of fresh fruit, and their freedom from tooth cavities is surprising.

MID-MORNING SLUMP

In a shop as huge as the Metropolitan's Home Office, with some 20,000 employees, many of them young girls recently out of high school, we are accustomed to a certain number of fainters. Some weeks, Dr. K. J. Thomson and his staff responsible for employee health, will see as many as twenty such cases.

No, it's not because they have been persuaded with a black-snake whip to "tote dat barge an' lift dat bale." Most of them never worked before, and seldom had to be anywhere on time, and they're not about to be pushed around by anyone now. They are mainly youngsters who eat no breakfast except perhaps juice and coffee. They'd rather sleep an extra ten minutes than have breakfast. By the latter part of the morning, their blood sugar gets so low that they feel weak and dizzy and sometimes faint. They are quickly revived with a little sugar by mouth and admonished hereafter to get up in time to eat a good breakfast. We always advise them to include some protein for breakfast such as eggs, milk, hot or concentrated cereal, or even a bit of meat.

THE PROTEIN BINDER

The reason for including protein in the breakfast is interesting, while we're on the subject of carbohydrates and sugars. Accurate measurements of the blood-sugar level show that immediately after ingestion of carbohydrates or sugars, that level rises markedly. But it recedes rapidly too and in an hour or two reaches a point even lower than it was before taking the sugar. If proteins are included with the sugar, however, the blood-sugar level rises and subsides much more slowly. In fact, it is pretty well sustained throughout the morning. It is as though the protein made the sugar more binding.

THE APPESTAT THEORY

This phenomenon, only recently discovered, gives rise to the "appestat" theory of hunger, so well described by Dr. Fred Stare of Harvard. It is of interest to those who are cowed by their appetite. Just as a thermostat automatically turns on the heat, the "appestat" turns on the hunger pangs.

The theory is that when the blood sugar gets low, hunger pangs commence. Thus a light breakfast—consisting mainly of carbohydrates—will cause an immediate incraese in blood sugar, but it doesn't last. There is a deficiency of blood sugar by mid-morning, with a resulting craving for a "coffee break" which usually includes 300 calories of doughnuts or a "Danish." This could conceivably reduce the appetite for lunch, but it doesn't seem to very often. If no coffee break is taken, then the appetite for lunch is considerable and one tends to overaet. If on the other hand, one eats a substantial breakfast including sufficient protein, the blood-sugar level is maintained throughout the morning, the appestat refrains from turning on the hunger pangs, and a light lunch is enough to satisfy.

One day I sat down to breakfast in the diner of a transcontinental train just as we were leaving a prairie cattle town. Into the diner came a heroic figure of a man, tall, tanned, lean, sixty-ish, with gray sideburns and the most beautiful handlebar mustaches I ever saw except on Buffalo Bill Cody. He was seated with deference by the steward, directly across from my table. Before ordering, he pulled a bottle out of his pocket in the tail of his long gray frock coat and poured himself half a tumbler full. It looked and smelled like whiskey. He downed it in a gulp followed by a few sips of water. And then, without looking at the menu, he ordered and ate such a breakfast that I jotted it down in my notebook, as follows:

1 whole grapefruit
Large bowl of oatmeal with cream and sugar
Large order of pancakes with much butter and syrup
Medium sized thick sirloin steak with butter
Cottage fried potatoes
Double sized slice of apple pie with ice cream
Six or eight cups of coffee with sugar and cream
(I lost count)

My breakfast companion, also a physician, whispered to me on the way out, "Well! To my professional eye that man looks healthy enough to live out the day at least, unless he dies of indigestion or accident." I'll still bet he wasn't hungry for lunch.

THE FATS

The third category of the basic foods are the fats. Quite necessary in moderate amounts to the well-rounded diet, they are highest per unit of weight in caloric value. Yet they are peculiarly satisfying to the appetite of the average American adult. Dr. Ancel Keys is convinced that the average American diet not only contains a higher percentage of fat than that of the several other countries he has studied, but that the percentage of fat consumed in this country has increased steadily over recent years. It appears to be true that the beef growers in this country have found better sale for beef which is tender and marbled with fat.

THE FAT'S IN THE FIRE

There is no question about fats being high in calories for their weight. They should be kept to a minimum by those who are counting their calories. This is true of all fats and oils, including the vegetable fats which are especially high in nut meats, ripe olives and avocados. Despite this general agreement, there is a book entitled *Eat Fats and Grow Thin*, and a while back a medical officer of the DuPont Company published a high protein and fat diet which he recommended for those wishing to reduce. The theory here is that severe restriction of fats in the diet leaves the individual hungry, and that supplying the needed calories largely through fats will still allow sufficient reduction of calories from proteins and carbohydrates to reduce weight with less aggravation by hunger pangs.

It may be that the fats have an even greater effect on the "appestat" than do proteins. But there is another reason for reducing the animal fats in the diet for those who are overweight and developing more than their share of hardening of the arteries, as we shall see in a moment. In any event, the orthodox reducing diet is very sparing of fats because of their high caloric content, and because strangely enough the body is usually already well supplied with them since the unused carbohydrates and proteins are changed to fat and stored as such in various fat depots of the body, mainly in the mesentery of the abdomen and under the skin.

I remember one time seeing a good surgeon finish an abdominal operation on a very fat woman. There was a good four inches of pure fat tissue between the skin and the abdominal muscles. He was slicing off great rolls of it, almost like cutting blubber from a whale. Dissecting out some ten pounds of it, he remarked,

"I don't usually go in for cosmetic surgery of this kind, but this good lady begged me to do it, saying it would save her months of uncomfortable dieting."

"Won't it return?" asked the intern assisting.

"Sure it will," laughed the surgeon, "unless she learns to become satisfied with less food."

"Well," said the anesthetist, "she'll have a few weeks of peace without dieting during her convalescence anyway."

The patient had a good recovery and was so proud of her flat tummy that she determined to keep it that way.

The main controversy in medical circles about the fats in the diet arises from the fact that they are a chemical jungle, not yet fully explored. As with all jungles, it is easy to get lost among things that are unknown and unidentifiable. With the aid of the amazing new gas chromatograph which will identify and quantitate certain combinations of molecules in infinitesimal amounts, there is promise of faster progress in this field in the future.

IS CHOLESTEROL THE VILLAIN?

Cholesterol, one of the several liquid fats in the blood, has repeatedly been found in excessive amounts in the blood of those with arteriosclerosis. It is present in the plaques which appear in the lining of the arteries which are beginning to thicken. But cholesterol is also found in what we suppose is excessive amounts in the blood of people with no evidence of arterial degeneration. Blood cholesterol commonly runs much higher among the people of Holland and Denmark, where cream, butter and cheese comprise a large portion of the regular diet, and yet those countries have a lower death rate from arteriosclerotic heart disease than we.

Among our employees, we checked the blood cholesterol levels of several hundred who had had coronary attacks (ample evidence that they had some form of what we are calling here, hardening of the arteries) against an equal number of the same sex and age who had no evidence of arterial disease. We found no correlation between the two. In fact, if anything, the normals averaged a little more cholesterol in the blood than the abnormals. Nevertheless, I suppose many doctors feel justified in limiting the cholesterol intake of their patients with early arteriosclerosis, partly because it is the one blood-fat that we know quite a bit about. But it's a dull diet, I must admit.

The fact is, there are several other fats and fatty substances in the blood stream besides cholesterol. Some of them, or combinations of them may be more directly related to arterial degeneration than is cholesterol alone. We just don't know yet.

MUST WE CHANGE THE NATIONAL DIET?

Meanwhile, comes the startling discovery by some, verified by others, that the animal fats, including meat, lard, butter and cream but not including fish oils, are all hydrogenated or saturated fats, that is, all of their molecules have combined with all of the hydrogen atoms that they can take. This accounts for their being semi-solid at normal temperatures, and as the food people say "good spreaders" (as for bread and crackers) which greatly affects their marketability. Most of the vegetable fats, including cotton seed and corn, are unsaturated, that is they have not combined with all of the hydrogen atoms they could take up. This accounts for the fact that most of them are oils, or at least will melt at room temperature. They're not good spreaders, hence are used mainly for cooking and for salad dressings.

But here's the catch that may make this a very important discovery: there is some evidence, fully convincing to some, still regarded with skepticism by others, that when taken as food these unsaturated vegetable oils reduce the saturated fats in the body, including cholesterol and the substances found in the plaques lining the diseased arteries. The exciting question is: Would substitution of unsaturated vegetable fats for all saturated animal fats in the diet cure or prevent the hardening, thickening and occlusion of the arteries which now so beset us?

Some people think so, and go so far as to drink a couple of jiggers of safflower seed oil daily in the hope of dissolving the plaques in their arteries, meanwhile avoiding as much animal fat as possible. Others go to some expense to buy Emdee, one of the few butter substitutes which is almost completely unsaturated. Others buy butter substitutes which are advertised as unsaturated, but if you'll read the fine print you'll find they have been "partially hydrogenated" in order to make them solid enough to be good spreaders. That means they are partially saturated.

Well, as in other promising research of this kind, who can say how it will come out? Promising leads like this have fizzled out before. The National Heart Institute and the American Heart Association are financing long-term studies in this field in various parts of the country. We should have the answer in a few more years, providing the enormous funds needed for this kind of research continue to be available.

Just suppose it proves to be true, that vegetable oils substituted for animal fats will prevent the leading cause of death in this country, degeneration of the arteries. What a Herculean task to change our national eating habits! Next to the addictions, such as narcotics, eating habits are among the hardest to change. We had some experience with this in the armed forces. A great majority of the boys and girls, especially from the middlewest, were "meat and potato" people. They would have none of that "rabbit food"—salads and green vegetables.

Even the pellagra victims in the deep South were addicted to their corn bread and salt pork. They had no appetite for red meat and vegetables. Orientals cling to polished rice. They often decline unpolished rice even though they learn that it will save them from beri-beri. The Japanese may or may not have been persuaded to eat grasshoppers to remedy their lack of the B vitamins. I don't know.

What I do know from years of experience in health education is that if we set about to persuade Americans to eat only lean meat and to forego butter and cream, we've a job on our hands. And think of the counteroffensives of the food industries and the dairymen!

Meanwhile, and especially if you are concerned about your weight, it may be just as well to cut the visible fat off your meat and go easy on butter, cream and lard for shortening. Broiling is much preferred to frying. The fat that drips into the pan or burns in the charcoal can't clog your arteries.

Well, enough about the fats before we get dehydrogenated ourselves or suffer from fatty degeneration of the intellect. To the great credit of the food industries which support it, the Nutrition Foundation at 99 Park Avenue, New York, N. Y., under the skilled direction of one of the world's most distinguished nutrition scientists, Dr. Charles Glen King, is supporting numerous promising food research projects throughout the world, with the ultimate object of producing better, more nutritious, purer and more convenient food articles for the public. To their great credit they have recently organized a bureau of health education from which reliable advice may be obtained on foods and nutrition.

THE MINERALS

One final basic component of foods, often so small in amounts as to rival the vitamins, and perhaps of nearly equal significance to health, is the group of minerals. "Trace elements," they are often called, because of their minute quantities, yet the absence of a certain one in grazing land will cause cows to abort their calves, and the lack of another causes goiter in human beings. Derived, of course, from the soil or water nurturing the plants we eat, or absorbed by the animals we eat, which have eaten these plants, they include sodium, potassium, calcium, phosphorus, sulphur, iodine, iron, nickel, magnesium, manganese, fluorine, silicon, copper and others.

In general, the minerals are found in, or just beneath the skin of vegetables and fruits, so eating the skin of potatoes, apples, pears and the like is a good idea, providing they are well washed.

Minerals are largely dissolved in boiling water. Hence the advantage of steaming or pressure cooking in little or no water.

Soups are rich in minerals, especially if poultry or meat bones have been simmered in them. That's partly why the kindly custom for neighbor ladies to run over to a sick friend's house with the bowl of chicken broth or beef broth for the invalid is so beneficial. They would simmer the chicken or beef and bones on the back of the stove all day, then season and strain. Little did they know that they may have been restoring the electrolyte balance which was upset by the illness.

For the most part, we need not worry about many of the trace elements since foods deficient in them are pretty generally understood and not sent to market. Foods carrying them in excess are likewise well known and either unpalatable or unsalable.

SOME MINERALS OF SPECIAL INTEREST

A few minerals deserve a brief discussion either because they are subjects of current controversy, or because we want to know why the doctor prescribes one or forbids another.

The first is *sodium,* which in the form of the chloride, or common table salt, is found in so many foods that the individual put on a salt free diet is really very severely restricted. Such restriction is justified, however, in certain cases of high blood pressure because, for reasons as yet not clearly understood, the sodium ion, either in excess or in combination with other body chemicals, does seem to have something to do with blood pressure. There is no doubt that some people with this particular form of hypertension experience much relief when salt is withheld. Later, they may be able to use a salt substitute such as potassium salt without harm, and still later, they may recover completely when the body-fluid balance is restored and the other mineral electrolytes go back into normal balance.

The body is extremely sensitive to changes in the salt level of the blood, and it is a marvelous mechanism which keeps this level so constant. Too much will overload and irritate the kidneys, where most of its elimination takes place. Too little will cause the symptoms of heat exhaustion which is always disabling and occasionally fatal.

Before the Hoover Dam was started, the Six Companies were advised that they could not build this dam in the Arizona desert without importing coolie labor; that few Negroes and no white men could stand the heat of that blazing sun, frequently reaching 120 degrees. To their great credit, they tried it without importing laborers. But during the first year they were much concerned over the number of men who had to be hospitalized for heat exhaustion. About a score of them died that first year.

About that time the medical director of one of the great steel companies made an astute observation about heat exhaustion which was very common among his men who worked around the furnaces. It caused more disability than all other industrial diseases combined among this group of men, and hardly a year went by without one or more deaths.

In studying his records carefully, the doctor noticed that one gang attending one furnace never had a case of "heat stroke," as the men called it. Watching their techniques carefully, he noted that after the heat was drawn, that is, the molten metal drawn off from the bottom of the Bessemer, and the men had a breather before the next furnace was ready for drawing, they all went across the street and had a beer, preceded and followed by handfuls of pretzels or salted peanuts.

It was known that copious amounts of salt and water were lost from the body through the perspiration. Could it be that these men were "sweating out" their salt and restoring it and their fluid balance with the beer and pretzels? Could excessive loss of salt in the blood be the cause of "heat stroke"?

To make a long story short, it was. Thus, the good doctor introduced the use of salt tablets and plenty of cool water for the use of all furnace gangs. Heat stroke was licked! Salt tablets and water boys were introduced at the Hoover Dam, and there were no more deaths and very few cases of heat exhaustion thereafter.

Thus we began to learn that loss of normal balance of sodium, potassium and some of the other electrolytes in the body fluids is a serious matter. This imbalance may occur not alone from heavy work in excessive heat, producing excessive sweating, but also from high fever in infections such as pneumonia or infantile paralysis; from extensive surgery; and from various diseases which disturb the usual normal balance. Few people realize what a boon this new knowledge has been to convalescence. Many people recover from serious illness today in one third the time it took only a few years ago because imbalance of the minerals in their bodies is now quickly detected and remedied.

Potassium is likewise an important mineral in the body tissues, acting in many respects like sodium, but we don't ordinarily have to be concerned with it in our diet. It is generally present in many of our vegetables and fruits and we seldom encounter excesses or deficiencies in normal people.

Calcium is required by the body, especially the bones and teeth, in considerable amounts and can rather easily become deficient in certain restricted diets, especially with insufficient milk intake. For some reason it is not easily absorbed when given in pill form by mouth. When milk cannot be taken, a good substitute is found in the harder cheeses, cottage cheese, bones and gristle, the latter being extracted by simmering for soups.

Iodine is of interest in the "goiter belts" of the country where it is deficient in the soil and water. Lack of iodine causes the thyroid gland in the front of the neck to enlarge, trying to mobilize for the body's use what small amounts are available. The soils of the mid-northern and mid-northwestern states of this country are notably deficient in iodine. In the coastal states it is plentiful, emanating largely from the sea.

Goiter cases were very common in our practice in northwestern Iowa. Most of them were benign and caused little concern except for the cosmetic effects among the girls. But every now and then one became "toxic," requiring prolonged treatment followed by removal of most of the thyroid gland.

Since iodized table salt has come into common use, this type of goiter has practically disappeared. And what a fuss the "antis" made over the addition of an infinitesimal amount of iodine in table salt! They were finally placated when it was pointed out that they could still obtain plain salt at the grocers. Nowadays, most people use iodized table salt, and no one thinks anything of it.

Iron is a necessary constituent of hemoglobin in the blood. Lack of sufficient amounts of it in the diet is thought to produce a simple form of anemia which is easily remedied by a tonic or pill containing infinitesimal amounts of iron. Some physicians prefer to give it hypodermically, or in combination with vitamins. Its excess in the soil or water is not known to do any harm, but it is sometimes troublesome, because it changes the color and sometimes the flavor of the water, tea, coffee, and whiskey.

Friends of ours built a beautiful little summer cottage over an iron-bearing soil in New England. Hoping to economize, they decided to use the water from their newly dug well without filtering or other treatment. At their housewarming, those guests who preferred "bourbon and branch" found themselves holding what looked like a glass of diluted ink. Whiskey turns iron-bearing water black. Such is the effect of iron on whiskey, neither of them harmful in moderate quantities, but having certain aesthetic disadvantages.

Fluorine is really a gas, related to chlorine and bromine, but usually handled dietetically, at least, as sodium fluoride. This is that controversial "rat poison" recommended by health authorities as an addition to drinking water to prevent tooth decay. Never have I seen such a furor kicked up by the "antis" over so simple a matter! And I bear many scars from past battles with the antivivisectionists, the anti-vaccinationists, the "natural foods" faddists and a host of others who can't recognize a fact when they see it.

Fluorine, usually in combination with sodium or silicon, is a natural ingredient of drinking water. It is as necessary as calcium in the bones, though in much smaller amounts. In those several areas of the country where sodium fluoride is present in the natural waters to the extent of 2 to 4 parts per million, there is a notable decrease in the occurrence of tooth decay among children. In a few places where sodium fluoride exceeds 8 or 10 parts per million, "spotted enamel" occurs among children, but even here the teeth are remarkably resistant to decay.

Dental caries is our commonest dental health problem in this country today, particularly among children and young adults. It is estimated that if all the dentists in the country could be persuaded to take only children as patients and attended only to their current needs, it would take over ten years to catch up. Half of our population have lost four or more teeth by middle age, and more than half of our people sixty-five years of age and over are entirely without any natural teeth.

There is no question but what many parts of the country must use drinking water which is deficient in fluorine. By adding 2 parts per million of sodium (or other) fluoride to the public water supply many enlightened cities have reduced the dental decay among children by 50 per cent. This is amply proved first by comparing the incidence of dental decay in school children in comparable cities like Colorado Springs and Boulder, Colorado. Boulder, with almost no fluorine in its natural waters, has nearly twice as much dental decay as Colorado Springs, where the natural waters contain around 4 to 6 parts per million. Similar comparisons have been made in England with similar results.

The second proof, and even more convincing, is the experience of cities like Newburgh, N.Y., Grand Rapids, Mich., Cleveland and Pittsburgh and many others, which have been adding fluorides to their public water supply to bring it up to 2 parts per million and have had a marked reduction in dental decay among children, with no ill effects to others, any more than there have been ill effects in Colorado Springs, where there is no choice.

And yet, to hear the "antis" rave, against adding "rat poison" to the water supply is something! And they've succeeded thus far, even though they are in a very small minority, in forcing many city officials into withholding fluoridation. They pose as experts, which very few of them are, they distort the vital statistics of the city, they beat the drums and clash the cymbals, until the city fathers think they are indeed a whole army.

At a hearing before one of the civic organizations a year or more ago, New York City's Health Commissioner, Leona Baumgartner, one of the ablest public health officials in the world, had just finished her testimony favoring fluoridation, when a man opposed to it demanded to be heard. He carried on the usual sensationally untrue, all-heat-and-no-light dissertation. When he had finished the Commissioner asked the chairman if she might ask this man a question. The chairman readily assented, hoping for time to catch his breath and try to sort out the false from the true.

Addressing the witness, the Commissioner said quietly and in her usual pleasant manner,

"Would you mind telling us what else you are opposed to?"

That did it. It loosed the flood gates. He was opposed to the income tax and the sales tax; he didn't like the labor unions who were ruining the country; he objected to public school buses serving parochial schools. In fact, there was little he wasn't opposed to except motherhood and God.

HEALTH EDUCATION—"WAS IST?"

Well, such are the vagaries of the public mind and in a democracy such vagaries have their full sway. I'm too old a public servant to be surprised at any kind of new "movement" that comes along. Usually they are amusing. But there is nothing amusing about our children beginning to lose their teeth at age nine or ten and going right on losing them until they have none left at the prime of life—age sixty-five, when something can now be done about it.

What beats me, too, is the indifference to medical advice shown by so many of our public officials. And I sometimes detect a similar indifference to medical advice by some business executives. Political and business executives soon learn great respect for the engineer, the accountant, the lawyer and the architect. And they quickly learn to recognize those who are good and those who are poor. But a medical scientist who may have spent his life learning all there is to know about a certain subject, is often given less consideration than a pseudo-scientific quack with a glib tongue.

I hope to live to see the day when we can persuade the public to do what they should do for their health, and to do it because they have had the benefit of some education on the subject, not because they were persuaded by a dictator's methods, effective as these may often seem.

I recall when I was a special agent for the Minnesota State Department of Health, we had a smallpox outbreak up on the Iron Range. All we had to do to get the population vaccinated quickly was to notify the local representatives of the Oliver Mining Company, the Mayor, the School Superintendent and the clergy. Most of the people there had come to this country direct from Poland, Austria and Hungary. They came flocking into our clinics all day and all night. Never a question or an objection. The job was done in three days and three nights and there was no more smallpox.

On the other hand, if there was a smallpox scare, say in the East High School in Minneapolis, the school to which the so-called better families send their children, there would be a storm of anti-vaccination protest, and it would take us three weeks to get even two thirds of the school population vaccinated. The "Bohunks," as these good people on the Iron Range were called, were accustomed to authority and obeyed without question. The educationally privileged at East High were skeptical and not yet convinced (a) that it was smallpox, (b) that vaccination would prevent it, (c) that vaccination was safe. To be sure, those who did accept vaccination knew *why* they did it. The Bohunks didn't. Worrisome as the better educated group was to the health officer because they were misguided or misinformed, I think in retrospect I would prefer that group, though I didn't feel that way at the time.

Not long after World War II one of our professional organizations devoted to health education invited a group of West German health officers to attend their annual convention and discuss techniques of educating the public in health matters. Since their expenses were paid for them, they came, but with much skepticism. Before the sessions began, one of them remarked:

"Health education? Was ist dis health education? Ven ve vant our people to do something for improving their health, ve *order* dem to do it. Und dey do it!"

They must have learned something at that meeting because soon after there was organized an international society on health education, now thriving with members from twenty-five nations, among whom the West Germans are most active.

HOW DANGEROUS IS FALL-OUT?

Before concluding our discussion of the minerals, let's spend a few moments on radio-active fall-out which is associated with the rarer metals like *uranium* and *radium*. Presently the cause of much unnecessary concern to the public, it may some day lead to our near annihilation in case of atomic warfare.

Many of the commoner metals such as lead, silver, chromium, mercury and gold have a very slight radio-activity, so slight as to give us no concern.

I recall one instance, however, in which the minutest amounts of chromium were of grave financial concern to a thriving big ceramic manufacturer. This story also illustrates how hysterical the public mind may become over a matter which really is no cause for concern.

THE CASE OF THE ORANGE-RED VASE

A group of industrial physicians was visiting a large ceramic plant, primarily to see at first hand some workers who were said to have contracted silicosis in infancy. This is a progressive lung disease caused by inhalation of finely divided silica dust in the air. To contract it in infancy is an unusual situation in this country. But it was accounted for when we learned that following the usual custom of the English potters in the early days at this plant, the family worked as a unit around the potter's wheel. The family often included an infant in the mother's lap so that she could resume her share of earning the family income as soon as possible after the latest baby was born. Here the baby inhaled the same silica dust as the others, and of course developed silicosis long before being old enough to join the family labors. But that's another story.

While in the plant, we admired some beautiful vases of a peculiar orange-red color, a color so unique that some of us suspected what was coming. Said one of us,

"Do these beautiful vases have a good sale?"

The Superintendent, who was our guide, smiled ruefully, and said:

"You bet they did! But we've taken them all off the market. Those you see here will be given our friends who are not subject to hysteria."

I said, "Well, I don't think I have hysterics. I'd be glad to have one, even before you tell us what's the matter with them."

With that, the Superintendent brought out his Geiger counter. Holding it near one of the vases, it clicked away, at a rate far beyond the normal background level of atom-smashing-atom in the normal air. The Superintendent said,

"The rare and beautiful color you see here comes from a special blend of chromates and mercurates. That particular shade cannot be produced in any other way. But it has just enough radio-activity to excite the most sensitive level of the Geiger counter.

"With such counters coming into more general use, and with people becoming so sensitive about radio-activity, we thought it best to withdraw these from our dealers and take the loss, before someone discovered it, went wild, and gave us some bad sales publicity."

At this point, he turned away from the vase and brought the counter toward a small desk clock with a luminous dial. It clicked away at a great rate, much greater than that produced by the vase.

"You see," said the Superintendent, "they're as harmless as a luminous dial on your bedside alarm clock. But people are used to alarm clocks, and not to these vases."

Whereupon, he gave us each one of these beautiful vases and we were glad not to be judged hysterical.

In this era of nuclear fission, many things have become slightly radio-active, or we have discovered radio-activity where we never looked for it before. There is one old church built of a certain New England granite which is so radio-active that it is laughingly referred to by the experts as "the hot church," though it would harm no one to live in that building his whole life. Practically all steel used in our skyscrapers and bridges in recent years is radio-active.

The worst scare came when uranium fall-out was found to have produced radio-activity in some of the dairy herd pastures, and was found to be carried through their milk. Some vegetables and meats were found to be slightly radio-active. Sounded pretty bad, didn't it?

Well, now we can all calm down as far as fall-out is concerned, so long as it doesn't get any worse, and it won't under present controls, and in the absence of an all-out atomic war.

There is always some radio-activity in the atmosphere. This comes from the very occasional chance collisions between atoms in nature. This "cosmic background," as it is sometimes called, is exceedingly slight. It is measurably greater at higher altitudes than at sea level. Yet there is not the slightest evidence that populations living at high altitudes are affected in any way whatsoever by this particular phenomenon of nature. In fact, Denver at 5,000 feet and Colorado Springs at a little over 6,000 feet are well known health resorts. Climax-Molybdenum operated enormous mines at over 10,000 feet with no ill effects from radio-activity on the workers or their families. The workers in the highest mines in the Andes, some of them over 15,000 feet, have no ill effects from cosmic radiation, though, born and raised there, they develop big chests and lungs.

In a word, we can all stand a lot more radiation than we normally get in an average lifetime without ill effects. But we do appreciate now for the first time, that there is a normal limit of radiation to which the body should be exposed. Radiation accumulates in the body. It is never eliminated. That is why doctors, dentists and other users of X-ray equipment and radium are now being careful to use only the safest equipment, and to give their patients only the minimum exposure to obtain necessary and satisfactory results. In particular, we try to avoid X-raying the pelvis of a pregnant woman during the first three months especially since embryonic tissue is more sensitive to radiation.

The radio-active metals won't harm you under ordinary circumstances.

THE DANGERS OF OVERWEIGHT

Before closing this chapter on foods and nutrition, just a few words more about overweight and its effect on health and longevity.

My colleagues and I in the Health and Welfare Division of the Metropolitan Life Insurance Company have been accused of making more men hungry than any others in the world. It's true, we had a lot to do with arousing public interest in weight control. This started in 1936 following one of a series of medico-actuarial studies which showed excessive mortality among people who were overweight. In these studies, the mortality experience of many life insurance companies with respect to certain physical defects is pooled. They often result in our being able to issue life insurance at standard cost to applicants with certain physical defects who were formerly charged an extra premium.

An example is underweight. Formerly these were charged more because early studies showed that, as a group, they had a high mortality. With the huge reduction in mortality from tuberculosis and pneumonia, most of them now get standard rates because the medico-actuarial studies show they now have a favorable mortality. Sometimes, conversely, these studies result in rating up people with certain defects or combinations of defects, because the latest experience shows this group to have unfavorable mortality.

So it is with overweights. There is no question that, as a group, they show more deaths at younger ages than those of normal weight. And the greater their degree of overweight, the higher goes their mortality. Most of the deaths are due to degenerative diseases of the heart, blood vessels and kidneys. There can be no question about this. Furthermore, overweight people who reduce their weight to what it should be, as a group, will revert to near normal mortality.

PAY YOUR MONEY AND TAKE YOUR CHOICE

So you pays your money and takes your choice. Do you want years of life, or do you want excessive food? It would seem as though you can't have both. (I say "seem as though" for reasons given below.) You can't fool the actuaries on this kind of thing. They know that 100,000 men all age thirty-five who are 20 per cent overweight will have many more deaths during the next fifty years than 100,000 men of the same age who are not overweight.

Hence, all this whoop-de-do, as some call it, about weight control. People who keep their weight within normal limits are likely to live longer.

IT'S MY GLANDS, DOCTOR

Say what you will about glandular disturbances, heredity, and other factors beyond your control accounting for your excessive weight. The fact remains that the vast majority of people are overweight because they eat too much. Those who would blame heredity usually come from a whole family of "sturdy folks" and "hearty eaters." "Sturdy" my eye! Just squeeze that upper arm. Is that sturdy muscle and "big bones" as they'd like to believe, or is it soft, flabby fat? Take a handful of that pot over the belly. Is that the tough muscle fibers of the circus strong-man, or is it just blubber? Fat accumulates under the skin, chin and chest when more calories are stoked into the body fires than can be burned, hence they're stored. Even those whose hormone-producing "glands" are at fault are few and far between, and even if the doctor succeeds in getting their glands back into balance they'll never attain normal weight until they stop eating so much.

FOR THE BIRDS

Of course, there do seem to be some people who can eat all they want and their weight remains stable. These are the lucky ones.

There are others who say they "eat like a bird" but everything they eat goes to fat. They eat like a bird, all right. Birds eat the equivalent of their body weight each day. And you'll find that most of these people, if they will keep an accurate count of their caloric intake for a few days, are really trying to emulate a bird.

WATCH THAT TUB, BUB

The vast majority of overweight people begin to get that way in their late twenty's and early thirty's. They are still stoking their body furnace with the amount of food they ate while finishing their growth and while fairly active. Now they have usually settled into a much more sedentary life. They don't need so much food, but fail to realize it.

That's the time to prevent overweight—when you notice the first ten-pound gain. It's easy to take off ten pounds and hold it. If you don't do it then, it goes on accumulating. Even a gain of ten pounds a year will put you fifty pounds overweight in five years. And then you do have a job getting rid of it.

I once helped a patient reduce from 320 to 190 pounds. What with backsliding from time to time, it took him a year to do it. But he really suffered because he'd been stuffing himself for forty years, since he was fifteen. And how he loved his food! But with 130 pounds off his bony framework, which was really rather slight, he was a different man—physically, mentally and cosmetically. He was convinced that had he started when he was twenty to hold his weight as of that age, he would have been much healthier, happier and would have been promoted faster.

SURE YOU CAN DO IT

Overeating is another of the addictions connected with food habits. Any addiction is hard to break, harder for some than for others. But it can be done and it will pay off. Be sure to see your doctor and let him prescribe the diet and the rate at which it is safe for you to reduce. In general, you can save much discomfort by seeking low-calorie, bulky foods such as cabbage, lettuce, cooked green vegetables and fresh fruits, with relatively larger amounts of protein, and *very* low amounts of sweet carbohydrates and fats. In only a few weeks, if you stick right by it, your "stomach will shrink," as they say, and the hunger pangs will subside. From then on, if you don't backslide and "stretch" the stomach again, you will be satisfied with smaller amounts of food for the rest of your life.

TWO CHEERFUL GUESSES FOR OVERWEIGHT

And now, I'll let you in on two conjectures, which may be of cheer. Bear in mind, they are only conjectures, based upon two of my "hunches." They may be wrong. (They usually are at the race track.) But anyway, they're for some of the poor old fatties to think about.

The first is about alcohol; not beer, ale, wine, whiskey, gin and vodka—just plain ethyl alcohol for beverage purposes. And I can see the frowns and headshaking of many of the nutrition scientists, and many of my medical colleagues and my prohibitionist friends when I spring this one. But remember, it's just a hunch. I could be wrong, and often am. Anyway, here goes:

Alcohol is extremely high in calories, as everyone knows. Most people on a reducing diet are advised to forego alcohol in any form unless they want to cut their nourishing food by an equal number of calories. One of my friends says, "I'd rather use saccharine in my coffee so I can have a highball before dinner."

I know of no scientific evidence that alcohol *per se* accumulates in the body in the form of fat. We know that it is eliminated, after going through the liver (where it may do some damage to some people), largely through the expired air of the lungs, and through the kidneys. But if I read my books right, it's all eventually eliminated. It does not of itself produce fat tissue.

It is rare to see a confirmed alcoholic who is overweight. The beer drinkers, sure, and sometimes, the wine bibbers, but they are rarely true alcoholics from a medical standpoint. I know a "wino" as they call them in the police drunk tanks, is the worst kind of drunk, but they're not bibbers (one who takes moderate amounts of wine with meals and occasional sips through the day.)

But I'm talking about alcohol *per se*. It does not store fat tissue in the body as do excesses of all other foods.

Therefore, it is my daring hunch, that a highball or "on the rocks" drink of whiskey, gin or vodka, will *of itself* not increase your weight. It will, of course, if you add a sweetened mixer such as ginger ale. Then you're taking in sugar calories. But you can't blame the whiskey. Beers and ales contain carbohydrates and protein calories from the malt which are considerable. Wines, even the dry ones, contain considerable sugar calories. They *will* have to be charged up to your surplus calorie account. Providing you can be satisfied with ice, plain water or plain soda for a mixer, I doubt if you have to charge up the extra calories in whiskey, gin or vodka, even though we know they're there. My hunch is—they don't produce fat.

Now to be sure, there are side-effects to the preprandial drink which some think are inevitable. They are not, if you guard against them. Alcohol stimulates the appetite, partly because it produces quick energy. So normally you will tend to eat more after a drink. But you can avoid this, if you haven't had too many to destroy your will power. And those canapes! How luscious they are, and just at the right time when you feel the hungriest! Count the calories in them, my friend! You'll be astounded, but don't blame it on the whiskey. If you must have a "blotter," stick to the carrot sticks and plain celery and rye-crisp.

I shall have more to say about the "evils of demon rum," as well as its blessings. But this much is just to give what cheer and encouragement I can to my overweight friends who, you'll admit, have taken quite a panning in this chapter.

The other conjecture, or hunch, which may give cheerful promise to some of the overweights, if they only live long enough, is that we may eventually find that there *are* different kinds of overweight people.

You'll recall this "riding of the overweights" largely started with the life insurance actuaries and their medical advisers. They *know* that overweight people are poor risks for life insurance and must be charged extra because of their higher mortality *as a group*.

Well, the same was true of the underweights twenty-five to fifty years ago. The actuaries found they had excessive mortality then, and charged them extra rates or declined them.

As time went on, the doctors discovered that there were different kinds of underweight people. The large group that the actuaries put in the pigeonhole marked "underweight" contained a great many people whose thinness was due to tuberculosis. Their proportion within the group was so great as to drag down the record of the whole group.

As the doctors gradually improved their methods of detecting tuberculosis, and finally of curing it, the residue of the underweight group were tuberculosis free. They turned out to be pretty healthy people. According to the latest figures available they, as a group, live a little longer than others. So now they get life insurance at regular rates and no further questions asked.

It is just conceivable, and it's already strongly suspected by some of our best clinicians, that there are several kinds of overweight people. Some, but only some, of them will develop high blood pressure, arterial degeneration, apoplexy and kidney disease and die earlier than they should. We already distinguish "malignant" hypertension in which, for reasons unknown, the blood pressure increases steadily and markedly, year after year, resulting in early death. The other kind is "benign" hypertension, in which the blood pressure fluctuates from day to day, and even hour to hour, depending on whether the individual is under a strain or emotionally upset. We're learning not to be so concerned with this type of hypertension. It is often brought under control by reducing slight excesses in weight and cutting down the salt intake for a while.

What is the difference between these two kinds of people? We don't know yet, any more than we used to know how to diagnose and cure early tuberculosis. Maybe solution of some of the fascinating mysteries of fat metabolism will shed light on the question.

Anyway, there is just the possibility that the day will come when we can differentiate between the hypertensive overweight who is headed for trouble, and the natural overweight who really was just "born that way," as he says, but who is not headed for trouble. If so, he can go on his way rejoicing, eating what he likes, and trusting that he can develop and retain enough muscles to carry around what he likes to carry, and paying normal rates for his life insurance. Meanwhile, he might "*Skoal!*" with the Scandinavian aquavit, but not "*Prosit!*" with the German lager, with no canapes and no overeating.

CHAPTER 6

WHAT MAKES US TICK— NOT ALL BEER AND SKITTLES

Hickory, dickory, dock,
The mouse ran up the clock;
The clock struck one,
The mouse ran down,
Hickory, dickory, dock.

MICE in your belfry? As the old nursery rhyme shows, not so long as you keep striking. But someday that mainspring of life will run down and it won't take another rewinding. How to postpone that inevitable day by watching your health will be discussed in this chapter.

By this time we should have some insight into "what makes the executive (not Sammy) run." He is a man apart, not like other men. He is endowed with super qualities of vigor, drive, ambition and high intelligence.

Let's see what makes us tick; that is, what kind of physical machinery we have, and what care it needs. To do this we may have to refer briefly to some anatomy and physiology. But I promise you this will not be another lecture on college hygiene. We may well find that hygiene for the adult executive is a little different from that for the college student. We may also find that our understanding of anatomy and physiology has changed considerably with the years of astonishing research since we were in college.

BROTHERS UNDER THE SKIN

One of my freshman colleagues in medical school was assigned a female cadaver for our routine anatomical dissection. This was the only female cadaver in the three dissecting rooms. Some of us were curious to know how he felt about dissecting a female, so we asked him. I've always remembered his reply:

"Except for a few little trinkets in the pelvis, the female cadaver is the same as the male—same muscles, tendons, blood vessels, nerves and viscera. It's only before they become cadavers that they're really different."

So it is with the executive. Different from others as he really is in life, he has the same physical construction as anyone else. Even his brain, which has served him so exceptionally in life, is no larger, nor does it have any different convolutions than any other.

THE FRANTIC SEARCH FOR GOOD HEALTH

There are a number of good texts which clearly describe the body mechanisms and how to care for them in sickness and health. Among them are: *The Textbook of Healthful Living,* by H. S. Diehl (6th edition, McGraw-Hill, 1960); *Complete Medical Guide,* by Benjamin Miller (Simon and Shuster, 1960); and *Modern Home Medical Adviser,* by Morris Fishbein (Garden City Books, 1956).

In spite of these and other good books on maintaining health, there is still a rich variety of fads and fallacies about "healthful" living in general circulation and belief today. "Just the facts, Ma'am," to quote Sergeant Friday, is what you will get in this chapter. If you already know the facts, or if your mind is already made up and you don't want to be confused by facts, pass on to the next chapter.

INTAKE AND OUTPUT (ELIMINATION)

A Period for the Colon

There has been nothing much new on this subject since college hygiene days, except for one or two new concepts which deserve passing mention.

Old Doc Cook, our professor of hygiene and director of the gymnasium, probably gave more hygiene lectures to more men students than anyone else. Among other gems of wisdom and common sense, he handed us this one:

When nature calls,
Do not bluff her;
For if you do,
Your health will suffer.

But taking this to heart, together with similar sentiments preached throughout the country, seems to give some people a touch of neurosis. If they don't have a bowel movement every day at the same hour, their day is ruined and they scurry to the laxative market.

This market is equal to the vitamin market, and indeed has been booming for a much longer time. The amount of good money the American public pays regularly for laxatives is beyond belief.

Now the use of laxatives can easily become a habit, and their continued use only encourages a lazy colon to become lazier. The same is true with a daily enema and even frequent periodic "colonic flushes." This, together with the fact that the intestinal tract, especially the lower bowel or colon, loses some of its elasticity as we get older, may throw the past-middle-age-executive into a bad fix if he has the laxative habit. He has to take more and more, stronger and stronger laxatives, having more and more worry about the contents of his bowel the while. This can be a real distraction, interfering with concentration, judgment and equanimity.

The facts are, first, when nature calls at an inconvenient time, you can bluff her if necessary in most cases, providing you haven't taken some kind of liquid dynamite called a laxative, and providing you aren't having a case of "the Texas trots." Second, it is not absolutely essential to have a daily bowel movement at the same hour. Convenient, comfortable and healthy, it is. The habit should be cultivated, but it's not a matter of life and death. Some persons are quite healthy with a b.m. every three or four days.

Intestinal toxins don't poison your system, as some would have us believe, providing your doctor finds that you have a healthy intestinal tract with no diverticula, ulcers or partial obstruction. It's usually perfectly safe to let nature take her course with that remarkable rhythmic peristalsis she has furnished us. And it does no harm to tell nature to hold her horses occasionally, if you've slept late and must catch a train or make a speech at the hour when you would ordinarily be in the bathroom.

NATURE'S REMEDIES

If you do feel a bit tied up, the chances are you need only drink more water for a few days, double the amount you usually have. Have a filled glass and a carafe on your desk to remind you. The next best remedy is more fruits, especially those like figs, dates, pears, plums, apples and whole oranges. If that doesn't work, a low enema, or often a soap or glycerine suppository, may loosen things up and put you back on balance again. But don't forget the water cure comes first.

The night wind was howling from the northeast across the prairies, threatening to turn the sleet into snow, as the old Ford slithered from side to side of the road. Nobody but a doctor or clergyman would be out on a night like this. And the road wasn't congested with clergymen, I thought somewhat bitterly. It was a hurry call to a sick baby fourteen miles out, at three A.M.

The baby was sick all right and I was glad I made it. She was four months old. The abdomen was greatly distended and hard as a board. Even my cold fingers gently palpating that little belly did not interrupt or increase the continuous low, agonized moaning which the mother said had gone on for twenty-four hours. Damn these people, I thought, why didn't they bring the baby into the hospital three days ago! Nothing in the diapers for four days but vomiting for two days. Fever of 105. White blood cells quickly done with my portable microscope and counting chamber, 20,000. Acetone odor on the breath, natural from the dehydration of the fever. I decided it was a case of intussusception, where a portion of the bowel telescopes upon itself, soon becoming gangrenous and usually fatal unless operated upon quickly.

It was a tricky diagnosis to make with no more facilities than those at hand. But if it was right, it would be trickier still to treat in that isolated farmhouse with no anesthetist, no nurse, and no instruments but those in my case. Besides, I had never operated on a baby alone, without assistance.

What to do? Take her to the hospital? I'd been taught these cases must not be transported except for very short distances in a carefully driven ambulance. The jolting might cause rupture of that little distended bowel. Get a surgeon to come out posthaste, of course, and we'd operate right there on the kitchen table, kerosene lamp or no. So I gave the mother the task of putting the wash tub on the kitchen stove and starting to boil up all the spare sheets and towels she had in the house, while I went to the telephone.

The surgeon quickly got the picture. He was an old hand at country practice and a good surgeon. But I sometimes thought he would fiddle around with a case all day, then at midnight decide to operate, rousing the nurses, the anesthetist and me out of bed for a job that might last until dawn. This time, as it turned out, I was glad he decided to "fiddle around" a little bit.

He said,

"Bill, I've seen a lot of those baby cases, like this. Your diagnosis may be right. But I know these people. You can't trust the mother's history of the case. And I don't know about that new-fangled blood-counting machine of yours, especially out there where the light is bad and your hand may have shaken a little with that pipette.

"Still, you may be right, and I'll come at once after you do this.

"Cut a small suppository from the laundry soap. It's purer than toilet soap. Insert the suppository, wait fifteen minutes, then put in a small amount of water with a hand syringe, slowly and gently.

"If that doesn't bring results, call me again and I'll be right out."

Well, you should have seen the results. No, I'm glad you didn't. I didn't know a little baby's bowel could contain so much.

I phoned the surgeon who laughed and said, "You don't need me." In an hour the baby was asleep, the abdomen was soft and the fever was down.

I said to myself, "A pretty fancy diagnosis, doctor. You just overlooked the fact that it might be just plain old constipation." And he was right about the inaccuracy of the mother's history. It was ten days of "nothing in the diapers," not four.

I cite this story to show you how I learned a healthy respect for just plain constipation. You can get right sick with it. Not so sick as that baby, perhaps, because adults don't get dehydrated so quickly as infants. But if you really have bad constipation, the remedy is not in the store's amazing array of laxatives. Go see your doctor.

GUARDIANS OF PURITY (THE KIDNEYS AND THEIR INFLUENTIAL CONNECTIONS)

Ever had a backache? Well, chances are it's not your kidneys. You don't need "Moans Little Kidney Pills" to relieve it. Except for their surrounding capsule, the kidneys have few sensory nerve fibers. So try a little aspirin and see if it doesn't relieve that lumbago, or rheumatics, or muscle strain that may be causing your backache.

One of the Standard Operational Procedures in the rough-house medical fraternity initiation is to give the neophyte a couple of tablets of methylene blue. It is harmless in such small amounts. But the customary result is impressive. About six hours later, sudden loud screams issue from the toilet, and out runs the freshman, fly open, eyes popping out, calling for any doctor in the house to come see what's the matter with his kidneys. His urine is an alarming dark blue color.

So you see, pills can do things to your kidneys, but "kidney pills" won't cure your backache.

Ordinarily, we don't have to worry much about our kidneys, even though they are a delicate and vital mechanism, responsible for removing wastes from the blood stream. All we need to do is to keep them well flushed by drinking plenty of water. We can even get along very nicely without one kidney; but not without two. A complete stoppage of kidney function leads to uremic poisoning, and death ensues. That may be the reason why so many people get excited about their kidneys when it's usually something else that's wrong.

There isn't much you can do to prevent renal calculi, as those stones are called, but it's a comfort to know that they occur more frequently at the younger ages, and usually do not recur.

Two young Harvard professors were hospitalized in the same room, both with kidney stones. First one would groan with paroxysms of pain, then the other, keeping each other awake. As the second night wore on, one of them in the midst of his travail groaned out to the other, "Let him who is without sin cast the first stone." To be able to quote scripture in the midst of a renal colic greatly increased my respect for young Harvard professors.

THE ROCKY ROAD

Some people's kidneys, especially young men's, produce stones for reasons unknown. So long as they remain in the kidney they cause no discomfort and are rarely detected except occasionally by chance in an X-ray. But when the kidney casts them out into the funnel-like kidney pelvis and they start going down, or obstructing, the long tube to the bladder (called the ureter), then you've got a real pain. You're entitled to some screams of agony then, and to as much opiate as the doctor will give you. Usually the stones pass through into the bladder and out through the larger urethra, but they can give you a few bad days or weeks. If they don't pass, they must be removed surgically, and the sooner the better, because continued obstruction of the ureter will put the kidney out of commission for good.

Most supposed kidney trouble is really bladder trouble, and the commonest cause of bladder trouble in middle-aged males is an obstruction of the urethra caused by an enlarged prostate.

"DAT OL' DEBBIL," PROSTATE

The prostate gland is an oval-shaped, egg-sized mass of glandular and fibrous tissue which completely surrounds the urethra just below the bladder. It's function is mainly to furnish a carrying vehicle for the semen, though it has other less important functions. Its fluid empties into the urethra through numerous tiny holes. Through these holes or through the blood stream, it may become infected and we call this infection prostatitis.

Acute infection is usually easy to control with proper antibiotics. Chronic infection is very difficult to cure entirely, though there is nearly always some improvement with repeated massage through the rectum (not exactly a happy experience, though patients seem to get used to it) and irrigations of the bladder.

We are not sure whether the prostate enlarges because of a chronic infection, or the impaired circulation and increase of fibrous tissue that accompanies the aging process. But enlarge it does in a considerable percentage of men past fifty.

Enlargement of the prostate produces a sequence of symptoms which, if they persist, should be given attention. The first is usually difficulty in emptying the bladder. The urinary stream is diminished and keeps "dribbling," so that one seems never to be entirely through. And that's just the case. The bladder cannot empty itself completely, the individual has to go more frequently, often several times during the night, and the amount passed each time becomes smaller. As a result, there is a stagnant residue left in the bladder which may become infected, adding cystitis to the woes of prostatitis. Then you really do need a doctor—a good urologist usually—but you should have seen him long before.

Now every enlarged prostate does not have to be surgically removed, as many men fear. So there's no excuse and every advantage in seeing your physician promptly. Of course, if the enlargement persists and increases and the bladder residue is persistent, then the doctor may advise removal of the prostate. This is a relatively safe operation nowadays. It has no deleterious effect on sexual desire or performance.

Bear in mind, too, that the prostate is one of the commonest sites of cancer. That's the reason for one of the less pleasant experiences connected with your annual physical examination, the rectal examination. Nevertheless, every routine health examination after age forty-five should include this rectal examination.

Of course, many men have a little difficulty from time to time in starting a stream or in getting the bladder completely empty. Sometimes tension or impatience alone will be the cause. It is only when these things persist that medical attention is indicated.

During the earliest experiences with "weightlessness" in supersonic planes, the School of Aviation Medicine was asked to investigate the complaint of some pilots that they could not urinate during this period, a matter of some concern before we send a man to the moon. Pilots were given huge quantities of water before flight time and asked to do their best when they became weightless. Despite being water-logged, they said they couldn't do a thing. The physicians and psychologists were convinced that the cause was "psychic stricture" rather than the condition of weightlessness, since the flow from the bladder is in no way dependent upon gravity. The distended bladder presses, the sphincter opens by voluntary command, and the urine is squeezed out as water is squirted from a rubber bulb with a hole in it. Determined to demonstrate, the doctors and psychologists finally took weightless flights with the pilots, convinced them with a visible demonstration, and the problem was solved.

Actually there's no harm in a normal bladder being well filled before it's emptied. The reflex mechanism in the sacral plexus which squeezes the bladder while the sphincter is open works best on a full bladder. I mention this because some men get so concerned that they attempt to urinate twice as often as normal, and thus never get the benefit of the squeezing process nature has so cleverly arranged.

It is wise to realize as you get older that everything slows down somewhat. Give your bladder the extra time it needs. It is important to take all the time necessary to get a complete emptying. Otherwise the residue accumulates, the bladder enlarges and sags, and finally gets so that it never will empty completely, no matter how long you stand there.

EXERCISE

Not being particularly robust in my youth, irked because my 128 pounds worth of six feet two inches could not easily do some of the things my contemporaries did, being susceptible to colds and sinus trouble in cold weather, I decided that fresh air and exercise were man's worst enemies. I lived comfortably with as little of either as I could manage.

I was wrong about the exercise. (I still have reservations about cold fresh air.) But more exercise would have done me good. It might have staved off some of the aging processes which bother me now.

Last year, Dr. Paul Dudley White, the distinguished Boston cardiologist, joined some of us on a tour of the new Clinical Center in Bethesda, Maryland, where the Public Health Service is doing such remarkable research on human illness.

Great exponent of regular exercise that he is, still riding his bicycle regularly in his seventies, he suggested that instead of waiting for the elevators, we all walk up the stairs to the seventh floor. I lasted until the third floor and by that time was so far behind the others that I found it expedient to sneak off to the elevator. I was still puffing more than he was when we met.

REGULARITY AND MODERATION

Yes, there's no doubt about regular, moderate exercise being good for us. It's been pointed out that more men die of sudden coronary attacks while resting in bed than during exercise. We know now that exercise never harms a normal heart—but it has to be a *normal* heart. Any impairment of the heart excuses you from operating the snow shovel.

We have also learned to fear the stagnation in the blood stream which occurs when the body is at rest too long or too often. The impetus for completing the circulation of blood from left ventricle to arteries to capillaries to veins, to right ventricle to lungs and back to left ventricle, does not come solely from the heart. An appreciable portion of such impetus comes from contraction of the muscles which gently squeeze the veins whose valves assure blood flow in the right direction, i.e., toward the heart. Complete and prolonged relaxation of the muscles, therefore, allows the blood stream to slow down so that the formation of a clot is more likely to occur. Once formed, the clot increases in size until the advancing end reaches a larger vein where the flow is more rapid. A portion is swept off, and if it lodges in the heart, lungs or brain there's trouble. Fortunately, such circulatory accidents, particularly that bugaboo of the surgeons, pulmonary embolus, which sometimes caused sudden death in an otherwise perfect convalescence, are almost a thing of the past since early ambulation has become the order of the day.

The sedentary executive in particular, whose work is done mostly at his desk, benefits from regular, moderate exercise—and I mean just that: *regular* and *moderate*. I do not mean thirty-six holes of golf on a Saturday or Sunday only when the weather is good. Nor do I mean several sets of tennis on an occasional pleasant Saturday, with no exercise in between. And the time comes all too soon when you can no longer keep up with your boys in running the bases, in demonstrating that famous old quarterback sneak, or teaching them the manly art with the gloves.

Of course, the amount of exercise you take with advancing years all depends on what you're used to. I dare say Dr. Paul Dudley White could outstrip me on a bicycle, just as he did on the stairs. He's used to it.

A fraternity brother of mine who was a tennis champion in school, as was his wife, is now medical director of a large life insurance company. Though now past seventy, both of them still play two or three sets of tennis, once or twice a week, either indoors or out. He says they don't play as hard as they used to, or run for the wide ones, but they still enjoy it. His heart, and hers too, I expect, are as normal as they were in college.

Even a damaged heart will recover, especially from a not too severe coronary attack. I'll never forget my amazement in San Francisco one morning at a meeting of the American Heart Association. Up over the brow of one of its very steep hills, walking firmly on his two feet, came a good friend of mine, a New York doctor, now well past seventy-five. Two years before he had had a fairly severe coronary attack. But here he was, fresh as a daisy, puffing very little. I lived in San Francisco for thirty years and gladly paid fifteen cents to ride the cable car rather than climb that hill.

WOULD YOU LIKE TO TAKE A WALK?

The seventy-year-old bicycle riders and tennis players are the exception, though. For the average business executive, walking—regularly and daily—is one of the most beneficial forms of exercise.

Among the advantages of walking is that one may set his own pace. There's equal virtue in a three-mile-an-hour clip, or an easy-going stroll. Both are rhythmic and bring into play most of the muscles of the trunk, back and legs. It's this rhythmic massage of the venous blood flow that prevents stagnation both of mind and body.

DO IT YOURSELF?

There is great virtue in golf for the same physiological reasons, and it brings the added zest of competition. It is good exercise for the elderly, even if they use the electric cart. The only serious disadvantage in golf is that some men tackle the game with the same passion of a Roman charioteer—to win or die. To play any game with every muscle tensed, jaw set and that old college spirit flaming is not exactly relaxation for men past their youth. Nor is it good for the high blood pressure too many of them have.

Swimming is excellent exercise for the executive, but it must be regular, two or three times a week.

Handball and squash are good for the younger executive, providing he's accustomed to it and doesn't think that the fate of the universe depends on his winning.

Massage, rubdowns and other passive exercise are better than none, but not so good as something active. A *moderate* work-out in a gymnasium if done regularly and at least twice a week is fine, but it's easily overdone. And, of course, one of the best, although least popular, forms of exercise is a regular set of calisthenics for fifteen minutes daily at home.

IS IT ALL CHEMISTRY?

Exercise has another function. The male hormones invariably produce aggressiveness. That's what they're for. And then there's adrenin, the old "fight or flight" hormone we met in Chapter 4. Some men have more hormones and therefore more aggressiveness than others. Over-aggressiveness can lead either to brilliant success or to seething frustration. In modern society, an excess of adrenin and other hormones producing aggressiveness can be a handicap instead of a life-saver. It's much better to work them off with regular exercise than to blow your top, or take out your frustration on your subordinates, or develop high blood pressure.

Just remember, with respect to exercise, you can't help slowing down as you age. Don't slow down any more than you have to, but don't drive yourself beyond reasonable limits. As with so many other things in a long and happy life, MODERATION is the watch-word.

REST AND SLEEP

When people grow older, their circulatory system sags a bit. Being in an upright or even a sitting position sixteen hours out of twenty-four, and not very active, the blood tends to "settle" in the dependent parts—abdomen, rectum, thighs, feet and ankles. This can cause real but unrecognized fatigue.

Dr. Oliver Wendell Holmes, Sr., (father of the late Justice Holmes) was Professor of Anatomy at Harvard, where his lectures were very popular. When demonstrating the bony structure of the human pelvis he would point to the two great bottom bones which bear the body's weight in a sitting posture and say: "These, gentlemen, are the tuberosities of the ischia, on which man was designed to sit and survey the works of Creation."*

Some executives sit too long at a time surveying the works of creation. Among the few physical defects more common in executives than in others are low back pain and hemorrhoids.

ASLEEP AT THE SWITCH? WHY NOT?

As sedentary executives get older, or develop some circulatory impairment, they get a surprising amount of relief and rejuvenation by "stretching out" for just fifteen or twenty minutes once or twice a day. There is nothing better for this purpose than a reclining chair which fits the contours of the body and elevates the feet and legs to the same level as the heart.

If I had full authority over the aging executives in a company, I could easily identify several of them with this kind of fatigue, and I would order for their offices a reclining chair of this kind, with instructions to shut their door, have phone calls held, and stretch out for twenty minutes right after lunch each day. They would get more done, do it better and live longer. The only precaution would be to have their secretary call them in twenty minutes, for before they know it, they'd go sound asleep within three minutes—and that's a good thing too. After all, an aging executive is neither a train dispatcher, nor is he on sentry duty, although some executives like to think they are.

Sleep habits often change as we grow older, and that's not surprising, nor is it anything to be concerned about.

I recall one sixty-year-old complaining to a contemporary that he couldn't sleep late mornings any more, awoke at five and wouldn't get back to sleep again. Said his friend:

"Yes, Charlie, I have the same trouble, but I don't mind it. Once you pass fifty you realize that your life is more than half

---

* Bowen, Catherine Drinker, *Yankee from Olympus*. Boston: Little Brown and Company, 1943, p. 108.

over. You don't want to miss any of what's left. So you wake early in the morning to see what's going on."

As the years roll on, many people tend to sleep less and to snatch little cat-naps during the day. When the board meeting is dull and the chairman speaks to them, they wake with a start and say, "Just resting my eyes, Mr. Chairman. Heard every word you said." And they don't miss much either. They've reached the age when many situations, new to the younger men, are much like the ones they've been through before. They know the answer, so don't worry about it until the youngsters find out what it's all about.

Sleep patterns vary greatly with different people, all the way from those like Edison who seldom slept more than four hours at a time, to the near narcoleptic who drops off to sleep on any and every possible occasion. Generally speaking, it is best not to worry about, or try to change too radically the sleep patterns of a lifetime.

COMMUTING

I am often asked whether an executive's health is better if he lives in the city somewhere near his office, or in a suburb which requires substantial time in travel every day. My reply is that what you do matters less than how you do it, and how you feel about what you're doing.

COMMUTERS, SWEET AND SOUR

If your commuting train has you enslaved, if you nearly have to break your neck to make it morning and night, if you're greatly annoyed by the inevitable delays and disruptions of service, then think it over. If, on the other hand, you can usually get a seat, have time to concentrate quietly on some unfinished business in your brief case, or read the paper, even do the crossword puzzle, then commuting isn't hurting you.

At one time I had a commute that took an hour and forty minutes from home to office. It gave me a chance to make some interesting observations on different reactions to commuting.

One group of four men always took the same double seat and

played a hilarious game of bridge both ways. One of them was selected to get to the station first and hold the seats. They kept a running score and had more fun over that bridge game than some of us had shooting craps in the army. It was a little club, and to them the rattling train and the lap board seemed to be as pleasant as a card table at the Union League Club. They would have missed commuting as a pleasant recreation.

One evening at a New York hotel bar I noticed five young men having their pre-train cocktails together and couldn't help overhearing their heated discussion. Each was trying to outdo the other in reciting the shortcomings of their respective supervisors in a nearby office. After a drink apiece they went to their trains. I asked the bartender about them. He said:

"Yep, that same bunch comes in every night before train time and gripes to beat hell about their bosses. Does 'em good, too. And think what it does for their wives. They get it off their chests here and spare her all that guff."

I'm sure commuting wasn't hurting them.

On the other hand, one particularly irritable and irritating newcomer to our train started cursing the railroad the minute he hit the platform in the morning. He fussed and fumed to all and sundry. Finally, one joker said to him:

"Well, why don't you tell the president of the railroad some of these things. He rides this train, you know."

"Does he?" exclaimed the irate one. "Point him out to me, will you?"

"Sure," said the joker. "You see that old man there with the full beard and the cane? That's him."

As the train pulled in the crank shoved himself into the seat next to the old man. For forty-five minutes he gave forth a steady stream of invective concerning the shortcomings of the railroad. Finally the gray beard reached over and took his haranguer's newspaper and wrote on the margin what we knew he would: "I am stone deaf." This little episode hardly made commuting any pleasanter for the irritable one.

So, commuting is like many other things in life. You take it your stride and enjoy as much as you can of it. If it gets you down, you'd better think about moving into town.

VISION AND HEARING

Occasionally one sees a person in his eighties able to read newsprint without glasses. How fortunate he is, but how rare. Most of us, as we get older, lose some of the elasticity in the lens and the ciliary apparatus of the eye, and find it harder and harder to focus clearly on near objects.

As one man at this stage said: "I can read anything without glasses. It's just that my arms aren't long enough."

There's nothing abnormal about this loss of elasticity in eyes—or arms. It's the inevitable result of the years. The only abnormality is resisting the necessity for glasses.

If You Need Glasses

It is always best to go to an opthalmologist, that is, an M.D. who specializes in the eyes, at least for the first examination. The reason for this is that there may be things wrong with vision other than aging; and sometimes an expert's examination of the eye-grounds, lens, and conjuctivae lead to the discovery of disorders elsewhere in the body which might be overlooked by one not trained in medicine.

Optometrists of today are well trained and skillful, and they know their limitations. Their skill is necessary in filling the doctor's prescription for just the right lenses to correct your vision, and in adjusting the new glasses so that the bows and frames fit exactly as they are supposed to. Badly fitting frames are almost as bad as the wrong correction in the lenses. After the initial examination by a physician, annual check-ups may be made by an optometrist if you wish. But there is a definite advantage to seeing an eye specialist at least every two years, whether glasses are worn or not. One important reason for this is to check for glaucoma, an eye disease which develops after age forty in most cases and which causes blindness if it isn't discovered and treated in time.

Hiding Your Hangover

The use of tinted lenses, and even "dark glasses" was much in vogue a few years ago, and may be so again. There are a few, but a very few, people whose eyes are so sensitive that normal daylight and artificial light needs to be filtered or cut down. With most people, however, tinted glasses tend to be a "crutch" and their continued use lessens ability to accommodate to extremes of brightness.

Many older people need dark glasses for extremes of light and glare, especially when driving, but they should be removed at once when entering a tunnel or when the sun goes down.

Hey, What Say?

As we grow older, our hearing, like our vision, often becomes impaired and for much the same reasons. The elasticity of the ear drum and its delicate activating mechanisms gradually lessens, and a "normal" type of deafness ensues, usually for the tones of higher pitch. Could it be that the aging ear just gets tired of all the screeching in life and deliberately shuts these sounds out in the interest of peace for the brain? Perhaps human hearing is becoming increasingly blunted by the roar of traffic and machinery, the wail of sirens and the din of crowds. Certainly there is a whole world of sound far beyond the hearing of modern man.

A tribe of aborigines, living in the jungle and seldom exposed to a sound louder than the swish of a wild bird, have recently had their hearing tested with the audiometer. The readings are said to be fantastic both in the breadth of the sound spectrum and in pitch and volume.

Zoologists tell us that there is no way to account for the amazing speed and agility of bats at night except through their extremely sensitive hearing. They emit continuous squeaks at a pitch so high that only a small part of the sound is heard by human beings. Like radar, they are guided in their swift flight by these sounds bouncing back from nearby objects. It seems incredible but the theory is born out by other animal observations.

Porpoises have been found to have a similar guiding mechanism.

They can be trained to follow an intricate underwater maze at a very rapid pace. Even with their eyes blindfolded, they will streak through an underwater course with speed almost equaling a skier's slalom, without so much as touching one of the markers. Apparently this is due to the bounce-back of high pitched sounds emitted continuously while the porpoises are swimming.

Hard of Hearing, Not Deaf

This is called presbycusis, as the aging impaired vision is called presbyopia. The victim is usually unaware of it, until it suddenly dawns on him how many people in recent years have taken to mumbling and he has to ask them to repeat. He also discovers for the first time how much easier it is to hear people when he can also watch their lips. This is the beginning of lip-reading which develops to a suprising extent even without the individual's awareness. It is one of nature's marvelous compensations.

At this point, the worker covered by workmen's compensation often gets an audiometer test. He is unduly impressed with his loss of hearing, runs to the compensation board and gets an award, claiming that his work-place has been exceptionally noisy and that the noise is what impaired his hearing. Probably half of these claims should be thrown out by the board because the man has nothing more than presbycusis due to aging. But in most jurisdictions, they get an award.

Unlike presbyopia, for which nothing connected with a man's work can be blamed, loss of hearing is sometimes caused by continuous and excessive noise. There's no doubt about that, as shown originally at Johns Hopkins and later in the Air Force. Thus, the employer who has not recognized an excessive noise area in some part of his shop, or if recognized, has done nothing about it, is often severely penalized by the attitude of these liberal compensation boards. They will attribute any hearing impairment to the man's work unless it can be proved otherwise.

How To Limit Disability

When even slight loss of hearing is first noted, that is the time to start investigating hearing aids and study lip reading. Many hearing aids are highly effective, but people must be trained to use them properly. Most failures are due to improper use and lack of training, or selection of the wrong kind of hearing aid rather than to the rare types of deafness in which none of them are helpful. They all magnify *all* sounds, including those our ear has learned during a lifetime to ignore. The rattle of a newspaper, or the tinkling of ice in a glass, can be frighteningly loud when first heard through a hearing aid. Training consists of learning to ignore these sounds as time goes on.

Deafness and Human Foibles

Perhaps the hardest part of the training is learning to adjust to the foibles of other people when they see someone wearing a hearing aid. Then, for the first time, it seems to the hard-of-hearing, they begin to speak loudly and distinctly. In fact, they begin to shout so loud that the magnified sound of their voice is actually painful to the ear. The hearing-aid wearer hastily reaches to turn the damned thing off and hear what he could have heard anyway if this idiot had only spoken clearly during the past few years. Then the shouter turns away so that his lips cannot be seen, and commences to shout at someone else, thinking to include the afflicted friend in the conversation. The other person answers in a normal voice. With his hearing aid turned off, the sufferer from presbycusis can't hear what was said. So it's no bed of roses, using a hearing aid, but the earlier one gets skilled at handling it, the more successful it is.

There is a great variety of hearing aids now on the market, some more conspicuous than others. Some are more effective for certain types of deafness than others. It takes a skilled otologist, and experienced hearing-aid technician, a co-operative patient and at times some trial and error to get the best results.

The Lonely One

If this early slight deafness is progressive, as it often is, though not always, the proper use of a well selected and fitted hearing aid may save you from developing a sense of loneliness and isolation such as very few other physical impairments ever produce.

People who have difficulty in hearing deserve more consideration than they usually get. Not hearing what the family and others are saying, they often tend to withdraw into a shell. Resenting this handicap which has been visited upon them, they sometimes sink into deep depression. Then, their hearing worsened by discouragement and lack of attention, they may stop trying to hear at all. Often they lose their sense of humor and become suspicious that others are talking about and ridiculing them. They end up making life a burden to themselves and everyone around them.

How To Help the Deafened

If you have someone in your family or office who is deafened, give him some thought. Think how differently we all seem to feel toward the blind. They automatically get our deep sympathy. The deafened person, on the other hand, automatically annoys us. When he asks us to repeat we do so in a sharp tone of impatience. Why is this? He can't help it. He craves the attention and participation he used to have. He hates to say, "What?" for fear of annoying you and exaggerating his disability. He will often pretend to hear rather than admit his deafness.

Make it a point to let him know what's going on. Sit down as near him as possible, face him and talk slowly and distinctly in as low a voice as possible. Wait to see if he comprehends and makes the normal response. If not, repeat more slowly and assure him you'll be glad to repeat a word he doesn't get. If this fails in a complicated business matter, tell him you'll explain it in a memorandum and do so. These people often compensate by learning to read and comprehend the written word very rapidly. One deafened friend of mine reads the equivalent of two books daily, one on his trip to the city, another on the way out, and he has developed a photographic memory.

From the Tragic to the Trivial

And now hear this. Not all impaired hearing is due to deterioration of the organs of hearing. Your hearing may be magically restored—in ten minutes!—by having the hardened wax washed out of your ears. But by your physician or an otologist, please. The delicate ear mechanism is no do-it-yourself area.

THE FUTURE, BETTER OR WORSE?

The unhappiest executive I know is the one who comes up to "retirement," as we call it, without having made any preparations. This is the man who has totally immersed himself in business all his life, with few outside interests. He will point with pride, and often justly so, that he has given the business a degree of devotion surpassing all others; that he has had more than most to do with the success of the business that he knows more of the employees and their values and weaknesses than anyone else, that he has more details of the business at his finger-tips than anyone else; and that the business would have gone on the rocks on this and that occasion if he hadn't done thus and so. He'll say: Golf, hobbies, civic betterment, church, recreation? When have I ever had time for such frivolities? He's always thought he was the one indispensable man.

Whether the years catch up with him through a compulsory retirement system, or he is forced to retire because of health, or a merger, or he's just plain fired—he's in trouble. No one man is indispensable in modern business today. If he is, he should have been fired long ago.

I recall the fate of one indispensable man of my acquaintance. He ran, and I mean *ran,* a huge, modern city department store. During the depression the store was in financial straits and had to be reorganized by its creditor bank. The first thing the new bank-appointed manager did was to fire this one indispensable man. He never recovered from the blow, and actually died of premature senility a few years later. But the store recovered, and today its business is thriving as never before. I must add that the remaining management of the store was almost as shocked as this poor fellow to find how nearly indispensable he was, and how much each of them had shucked off his responsibilities on to his shoulders. But it resulted in a real management, not a one-man show.

This is a peculiar form of super-egotism for which there is little call in modern times.

ALWAYS LOOK AHEAD

The modern executive realizes that his business cannot be everything in his life. He must deliberately plan his days and years so that he has time for his wife and family and for some interest in civic betterment for his community and nation; at least a little time and money to devote to those less fortunate; and still have time for himself to do some of the things he enjoys.

This is the kind of executive I never have to worry about. He's well-balanced, alert to what goes on around him, takes his business in his stride—a stride that matches the pace he has set for himself. He delegates authority and expects it to be lived up to. Eventually, and long before his normal retirement date comes, he finds satisfaction in so many interests that he begins to "taper off" in his business activities, turning more and more things over to his lieutenants and subordinates, being prudent about his personal financial status, so that he is more than ready to "graduate," not retire, from one kind of life to another which is attractive to him and promises even greater satisfactions than he has known.

RETIREMENT OR "GRADUATION"?

I often wish we could do away with the word "retirement." It has come to carry connotations of idleness, separation from pleasant life-long patterns, compulsory severance because of age—"too old to be any good any more." It should never mean any of those things, especially idleness. Most of those who are suddenly idle after years of activity, deteriorate rapidly. Of course, idleness to one man means something else to another.

I recall a dentist who did moderately well, owned his home and did not have an extravagant family. He was gracious about accepting a little financial help from other members of the family from time to time, especially as his two husky boys were growing up. But he made up his mind rather early in his professional career that he would retire from dental work in not more than thirty years. And he did retire at fifty-five.

He and his wife didn't have much to live on, and his boys, who had been rather easy-going with their earnings until then, were a little taken aback at his expectation of modest financial help from then on, though they had been amply warned. He settled back, pulled his favorite rocking chair into the bay window, spent the first two hours of each morning there reading, then did a few household chores, walked several blocks to his modest club where he played whist or billiards until mid-afternoon, walked home for a nap and more reading and visiting with cronies, had dinner and retired after his favorite radio broadcast. Neither he nor his wife ever wanted a television set. He's been following that same routine for twenty years. He's now seventy-five, hale and hearty and happy —good for another twenty-five years I'll bet.

Idle, you may call it, but it's what he wanted to do and he's happy at it. I doubt if he was ever really a business executive.

Most business executives, because of their superior intelligence, naturally develop broad interests and lead active, busy lives. They find great satisfaction in being busier than most and show an amazing capacity to interest themselves and become more or less proficient in many diverse fields. Because of their eminence in the business world they have many invitations to participate in various community activities. In fact their problem during their active years is not to spread themselves too thin. They must learn to decline gracefully many flattering and intriguing invitations. They blissfully think this or that invitation is "something I'd like to take an interest in when I retire.' "

Better pick up a few of them now, my friend, get familiar with the activity so that you may have the satisfaction of making worthwhile contributions to it while you're still active.

THREE FALLACIES

Three things that are almost axiomatic fool many of us. One is that you can't drop something that you've been doing with all your might, and enjoying immensely all your adult life, and pick up something else totally unrelated and expect to enjoy it equally. If you fool yourself into thinking that, you're in for disillusionment and your retirement will be unhappy. You're a novice in the new field and it will be a long time before you earn the skill and prominence in that field that you enjoyed in your earlier field. Much better begin developing knowledge and skills in the new field as a hobby to which you devote considerable recreational time for some years. Even golf or fishing or travel can be monotonous when you have nothing else to do.

The second is that the invitations to join this or that worthy enterprise will drop off amazingly when you're no longer an important company man. Unfortunately, all many of them wanted was your name on their letterhead, not your brains.

The third is that you will inevitably slow down, so that what looks now as though it would be interesting ten years hence, may prove altogether too strenuous for you then. By that time, the medics may be restricting your activities to your great disappointment because of a heart condition or stiffened joints, or something else. Anyway, it's just good sense to realize that the time will come, sooner or later, when you are just too old to do all the things you'd like to do in the way you thought you could do them. My suggestion is: keep going as long as you can; don't give up unless you have to; but when you have to, do it gracefully. Use the cart for nine holes of golf instead of scaring your partners with that apoplectic look over eighteen holes.

CONCLUSION

Looking back over these last two chapters, I've given you quite a slug. But I think some understanding of what makes us tick as we do, and why we don't tick so well at times, may be reassuring and helpful in everyday life.

These are mostly the things on which I'm questioned oftenest by executives. With many it is highly gratifying for me to see how quickly they understand even a difficult and complicated answer and seem to profit from it. With others, I'm dismayed at how little they know of the ordinary workings of the human machine and how hard it is to help them understand what's the matter with them.

Those who worry and sadden me the most are ones who figure "what you don't know won't hurt you." Never was there more fallacious reasoning. Ignorance is just what does hurt you the most often. They are so frightened over the least little thing wrong with them that they shy away from the doctor for fear he'll frighten them more. These are unhappy men, living in the caves of darkness so far as their health is concerned, and like the ancient caveman afraid of the sounds and smells which surround them with imaginary enemies threatening their destruction.

In this enlightened age with so much knowledge of what makes us tick and how to keep on ticking, it is no longer reasonable to be afraid of the doctor. His knowledge is willingly imparted and more often than not is reassuring and helpful.

Herein, I have tried to explain simply, and give helpful suggestions on, some of the more common disorders that assail us as we get older; and how to be prepared in some measure for the inexorable bodily changes brought on by the years. Were I to try to sum it all up in one word, that word would be:

MODERATION

CHAPTER 7

CALMER-DOWNERS AND PEPPER-UPPERS

Few animals aside from man are prone to keep doing things to make themselves feel different. Man alone deliberately keeps on swallowing, inhaling, even injecting, himself with substances to change his mood. He takes a poisonous plant, small portions of which give a cat fits, and either chews it, snuffs it or burns it to inhale the smoke—tobacco. He goes to some trouble to make drinkable a chemical poison, ethyl alcohol, and uses it as a beverage. He pays a handsome price for pills to put him to sleep, to wake him up, to calm his nerves or to stimulate his brain—"pep pills" and tranquilizers.

Isn't it funny when you stop to think of it? My little dog liked a lick or two of beer. Monkeys have been taught to smoke. Cattle go crazy if they eat loco weed, but that's really accidental poisoning. Generally speaking, however, animals other than man do not seek out an unnatural food or drink or inhalant, just to make them feel different.

ORIGIN OF SPIRITS

Whatever the reason for this pecularity, it has been with us almost from man's beginnings. Berton Roueché in an interesting series on alcohol in *The New Yorker* commencing January 9, 1960, quotes some prehistorians as believing that religion didn't begin until man stumbled over a mild intoxicant or narcotic which gave him strange dreams. Alcohols, ethers, or narcotics of some kind were very early associated with tribal religious ceremonies. According to Roueché all but three of the numerous Stone Age cultures "had an indigenous familiarity with alcohol." In fact, the tribal medicine men found out a lot about medicines and drugs of various kinds, and eventually passed this knowledge on to the pioneers of more respectable medicine.

As long as these magic potions remained solely in the hands of the doctors, witch or otherwise, they caused no more trouble than was planned—a wedding, or a defloration ceremony, frenzied dancing, or war on another tribe. But as soon as some of the people found out how to make various potions by home brew methods, there was trouble of another kind. This was the kind of trouble that led tribal leaders to think that something should be done about it. Then another social phenomenon, also almost as old as mankind, appeared—a prohibition bloc.

And so, almost as far back as human history goes, we've had the overindulgers on one side, and the makers-of-laws-against-any-indulging on the other side. Both groups are apparently here to stay, so let's look at some of the indulgers and what they indulge in. We'll let the prohibitors alone. They probably do more good than harm, as long as they're in the minority.

ENLIGHTENED INDULGENCE

Many years ago when scheduled flying time from coast to coast was twenty-one hours (and we seldom made it that quickly), I started a flight one night with a very able physician who taught pharmacology in his medical school. Like most of us, he had a briefcase full of work to do and a pocketful of pills. As soon as the seat belts were off, he stepped to the water cooler and washed down a couple of pills, then worked with great concentration for three hours. Then he had another sip of water and down went some more pills. In five minutes he was asleep and slept soundly for two hours. Then he was up for some more pills, wide awake, and worked another three hours. Pills again, and he slept a couple of hours. This went on the whole length of the journey.

When he seemed about through with this remarkable performance and we were circling for a landing at LaGuardia, I felt I knew him well enough to make inquiry, thinking to learn something. And I did.

He said, "Well, Doctor, when one knows the pharmacopoeia as well as I do, I see no reason for not using it to my advantage. I take a small dose of a caffeine derivative to make me wide awake until I get a certain amount of work done. Then I take a small dose of phenobarbital and sleep soundly for a couple of hours. That way, I help my system adapt to this unusual night and this unnatural mode of travel."

I have often thought that he had something there. He was not a drug addict. The carefully measured amounts of medication he took did him no harm. He had finished a lot of work and had had a reasonable amount of good sound sleep. He was brighter than I was at the meeting next day and didn't have the usual four o'clock fatigue that hits most of us who have been awake most of the night before. It may be rationalizing, but I like to think that is the way sensible and well-balanced people have learned to live with their "pepper-uppers and calmer-downers," which are so plentiful and relatively easily available to us today. They range all the way from tea and coffee to tobacco, alcohol and the opiates, the latter not so readily available, but having their place, nevertheless. When not abused, all these things really do make life easier for many people. It's their abuse which makes the trouble and fans the fires of the prohibitors.

INDIVIDUAL PECULIARITIES

Before we begin to discuss the real effects of these various stimulants and tranquilizers, let me make it clear that there are some individuals who should never touch one of them.

I had a patient who was greatly troubled with "hives" and occasional bouts with asthma. The hives would come out in great welts on his skin, and one could literally write on his back by the light stroke of a fingernail. The attacks came on at strange times, seemingly without rhyme or reason, and were really disabling for a day or two.

Eventually we found that he was sensitive to shell fish of all kinds. By eliminating them from his diet his difficulty disappeared. Once, he took just a spoonful of what he thought was cream of tomato soup. It was lobster bisque and he was up all night with hives again.

The important point here is that there are some people who simply cannot tolerate certain foods, drinks or drugs. Some can't eat strawberries, some can't drink milk, some have their digestion upset by beef, others are especially sensitive to aspirin, or coffee, or onions. One man I know can't tolerate morphine—makes him as sick as a cat—and did the surgeons have a merry time with him!

These are personal and individual idiosyncrasies, the causes of which give rise to much speculation. Are they truly hereditary or just the result of childhood suggestibility by a parent who virtually boasts about his idosyncrasies? Are they the product of some incident in infant feeding when the intestinal lining is not yet mature enough to sort out a great variety of new and strange proteins? Or are they just the result of some minor but peculiar imbalance in an individual's body chemistry? No one knows yet, for sure, but they certainly do exist. The sooner discovered and reckoned with, the better; and the person who ignores such sensitivities is very foolish indeed.

So it is that some people should never drink coffee. They are peculiarly sensitive to the caffeine, or perhaps some of the aromatic oils, and coffee gives them the jitters—nervousness, shakes and wakefulness. They won't get over it by ignoring it. Coffee is not for them, period. Some can't eat oysters, or clams, or pork, or what-have-you. And that's that. They just *must* stay away from whatever it is that makes them react differently from most people to a given food, drink or drug.

ALCOHOLIC BEVERAGES

Individual Reactions

This is especially true of alcohol. Some people are just not good drinkers, and they shouldn't try to be. They either get somnolent or noisy or belligerent on one or two drinks; or they got unco-ordinated, commence to spill things and stagger when they walk; or one drink sets them off and they can't stop until they're pie-eyed. They're the ones whose wives either become prohibitionists or, worse still, "defense" drinkers, trying to keep up, drink for drink, with their husbands. Often, it is the wife who becomes an alcoholic as a result, but usually both of them do. Alcohol is not for these people. It's their misfortune that one drink doesn't make them so sick as one oyster will make a person who is sensitive to oysters.

There is great variation in tolerance to alcohol with different people. Fortunate is he who has an "alcostat," some little signal in his brain which tells him when to stop, and wise is he who heeds it. Unfortunately, alcohol beyond a certain amount tends to lower the inhibitions, and the alcostat is too often ignored.

Often a Friend to Man

Apart from these two groups, the people who are supersensitive to alcohol and should never touch even a drop, and those whose natural tolerance is low, alcohol in its various forms has, on the whole, been a pretty good friend to man. He has lived with it for centuries and, in the main, has treated it with respect, using it as the pharmacology professor did his drugs to help his system adapt to the artificialities and vicissitudes of life.

Most sensible people know their limitations and seldom transgress them. According to the National Council on Alcoholism, about sixty-five million Americans use alcoholic beverages in some form. Of these, perhaps four million are excessive drinkers who may or may not become alcoholics. Those who have actually acquired the deficiency diseases of chronic alcoholism are estimated at about 800,000. These are of course only rough estimates but they help support my over-all statement that, in the main, alcohol is a friend to man.

This is no place for a complete dissertation on the virtues of alcohol in moderation, nor indeed for a lecture on the evil effects of demon rum. Anyone interested, and especially anyone concerned with a friend's drinking problem should read *Social Drinking—How to Enjoy Drinking Without Being Harmed by It,* by Dr. Giorgio Lolli, published in 1960 by the World Publishing Company of Cleveland and New York. I have watched Dr. Lolli's work with alcoholics and followed his thorough physiological as well as psychological studies on the effects of alcohol, and consider him an authority.

Some Advantages in the Preprandial Drink

Suffice it to say that in my opinion, based upon many years observation on the health of executives, the preprandial cocktail, and especially the well-diluted highball, is not harmful and is often beneficial for any man not unduly sensitive to alcohol. This goes for a drink before lunch, too, providing it doesn't dull the executive's finest judgment for the afternoon's work.

Cocktail vs. Highball vs. Wine or Beer

As for cocktail vs. highball, some stomach linings are more sensitive than others. If we all realized what a delicate and intricate apparatus this is, and how we depend upon it to absorb automatically those food elements we need, how it controls the amount and kind of digestive juices required by the sometimes surprising articles we eat, how it directs the muscles which churn and pass on our nourishment to other even more selective linings in the small intestine, we would think twice before insulting that sensitive membrane with a highly concentrated alcoholic drink which burns our tongue and throat.

I know the TV Westerns depict the sturdy cowboy or robber as drinking his whiskey neat. But I also judge from these Westerns that few of them lived long enough to enjoy middle-age, much less dyspepsia. Anyway, I personally favor considerable dilution either in the highball glass, or in the mouth and stomach by small, infrequent sips of a cocktail, giving the saliva and gastric juices a chance to dilute the caustic effect.

From the standpoint of avoiding insult to the digestive processes, many European drinking patterns are superior to ours because they call for food with drinking. Although wine with meals is considered a necessity in many countries, it is seldom preceded by a highball or cocktail. As the formal dinner courses are served, different kinds of wine are poured—sometimes in considerable quantities it is true—and the dinner winds up with a liqueur, usually brandy for the men. But at no time is the empty stomach assaulted with a concentrated irritant; the brain is not suddenly struck by liquid lightning, and the conversation is not disorganized by the searing impact of a straight "shot."

In the beer and ale drinking countries of Europe, also, people usually eat steadily while they drink. The alcohol is well diluted and capacity automatically limited by the quantity of liquid which must be absorbed. Again, the brain and digestive systems are not violently assaulted, and if the drinking is leisurely enough, the blood alcohol seems to reach a plateau at least as far as sensation is concerned. Physiologically, of course, inebriation sneaks up more slowly but just as inevitably if enough alcohol accumulates.

To mix the products of the vine or brewhouse with the products of the still is to court a headache for some people, for reasons not clearly understood. It may have something to do with differing rates of absorption.

Stimulant or Depressant?

Alcohol is considered a stimulant by most people, but classed as a depressant by physicians. Its main and first effect is to pull down the curtain on the forebrain, that is, to numb it. Both memory and fine judgment are among the first of the forebrain's functions to be affected. But so also are fears, worries, and inhibitions, the "tricks of the forebrain" often unmasked and dissipated. Now perhaps, that dull headache disappears, or that vague abdominal discomfort is gone, or that depressed feeling is relieved. As inhibitions fall away, we feel free, relaxed. Life looks brighter and well worth living. Imagination bubbles and ideas flow readily. (Just be sure you can check the ideas again before acting on them; they may not look so good tomorrow when judgment comes back.)

Four Facts about Alcohol

One thing to remember about liquor is that even one drink makes it harder, rather than easier to change your mood. Thus if you are really depressed, or angry or just plain cranky, a drink or two is likely to make you more so. Get your bad mood changed first.

Another thing to remember is that alcohol and gasoline don't mix. If you drink, don't drive.

A third thing to bear in mind is that the body labors long and mightily to get rid of alcohol. It appears in most of the cells of the body within moments after the first drink. It circulates largely unchanged in the blood stream, through the heart, brain and liver time after time after time, until finally it is broken down into carbon dioxide and water and blown out through the lungs. Dr. Lolli quotes Dr. Greenberg as showing that the alcohol in one highball or cocktail (1½ ounces) is not entirely eliminated for two hours, and five highballs of similar amount will take ten hours to eliminate.

Finally, among the things to remember about alcohol is that if you have a hangover, it's because you've had too much and the poor overworked body cells are still struggling with it, especially the liver, which has to detoxify it before the more respectable cells will even start breaking it down. The "hair of the dog" theory is a fallacy. An eye-opener may open your eyes, but it only adds insult to the injury of those cells which have been overworking while you slept and now will have to work some more because of the eye-opener. Outside the hospital, where intravenous therapy can be given, there is no cure for hangover except to sweat it out. A little exercise and some clam juice, or other food rich in the B vitamins may help.

Alcoholism in Industry—Worse Than Taxes

Every executive with a payroll of any size must be concerned about chronic alcoholism among his employees. Here is the cause of much excessive absenteeism, but more costly and less apparent is the bumbling inefficiency and undependability of the alcoholic. Alcoholism in industry occurs in from 2 to 4 per cent of all employees, depending on local customs and the type of industry. But the losses caused by these unfortunate people are far out of proportion to their number.

The discovery of an alcoholic and the necessity to do something about him, or her, frequently takes the executive by surprise, especially when he learns that this has been going on for years and he was never told about it. This is a peculiarity of alcoholism. Unlike any other condition of such seriousness, the individual is hidden by his associates who cover up for him and even do his work for him without reporting it. He is frequently a pleasant, outgoing individual with many friends who mistakenly think they are doing him a favor by protecting him from the wrath of management. Instead of friendship, this is often the kiss of death because unless he is rescued, the alcoholic is doomed to progressive deterioration, eventual loss of friends, loss of job, loss of family and early death.

More Than Half Are Curable

Much can be done for the alcoholic nowadays through medical and psychological means. One large industry reports a salvage rate of 90 per cent for those found fairly early, given modern medical treatment, and guided to Alcoholics Anonymous or some similar influence. A salvage rate of 60 per cent is fairly common in an enlightened industry.

To have any salvage rate at all, however, top management must indicate interest and concern and see that all those in supervisory positions take proper responsibility for helping to identify cases, referring them to a modern and well-equipped medical department. Without this personal and continued interest by management, the problem is never solved, and the business continues to suffer untold hidden losses. The National Council on Alcoholism in New York City and its several local affiliates over the country will furnish a number of carefully worked out and successful alcoholism programs in industry.

The Employer's Unique Advantages

The employer has unique advantages in helping control this growing national health problem. First, he is often the only one able to demonstrate to the individual a deterioration in work. This is quite apparent from absence records and errors.

Second, he can treat it not as a moral problem but just a straight business proposition: you can't afford to pay for carelessness and undependability; hence it must stop.

Third, it has been demonstrated time and again that the long-time employee values his job even more than he seems to value his family and friends. The prospect of losing that job is a sobering influence in more ways than one. But he must be brought face to face with that stark reality, and know by observation of action taken on others that the boss means it.

Fourth, industry, through its personnel and medical departments working together, can often persuade the alcoholic to do something about it more easily than anyone else because it is done objectively and impersonally, free of the emotional complications which handicap his family and friends.

The success of modern industrial programs in the control of alcoholism is an encouraging breakthrough on a serious national problem that has been most discouraging until now.

Moderation and Tolerance

Speaking generally, the successful executive has long ago made his peace with alcohol, or he wouldn't be where he is. My purpose here has been to try to clarify some misconceptions about its use in the hope of, on the one side, helping the executive who himself belongs to the "prohibitors" school of thought and needs to become a little more tolerant toward his subordinates who take an occasional drink; and on the other side, to allay the fears of those who indulge moderately but have been brought up to think that one drinks starts them on the road to perdition and so feel guilty about it. The guilt feeling probably does them more harm than the drink. Here again, as with exercise, tobacco, work and food, moderation is the watchword. To this with respect to alcohol, I would urge the executive to add tolerance toward others who may feel differently than he, at the same time dealing firmly with those whose excess drinking is leading them toward deterioration and early death.

TOBACCO

In March, 1961, France began a full year's observance of the introduction of tobacco four hundred years ago and the 150th anniversary of the Napoleonic decree establishing the Government tobacco monopoly. Nicotine, the active ingredient of tobacco, was named after Jean Nicot, French Ambassador to Portugal, who is credited with bringing the first tobacco in the form of snuff to the Regent Catherine de Medici four centuries ago. Sir Walter Raleigh might dispute this, but that is immaterial. We see, then, that tobacco is a relative newcomer to the list of man's addictive foibles, compared with the juice of the poppy producing opium, the analgesic Indian hemp, and the more potent poisons like hemlock and curare.

Sales and Taxes Increase

The sale of tobacco in this country continues to increase, year after year, especially in the form of cigarettes and cigars. Even snuff and chewing tobacco have held a remarkably steady market in recent years. Tobacco production is the mainstay of the agricultural economy in many of our states, and its production increases yearly despite ever-increasing taxes on the finished product.

Cigarettes and Lung Cancer

There is increasing evidence that the climbing death rate from lung cancer, especially among males, is associated with *excessive* cigarette smoking (two or more packs a day). Cigarettes are condemned by the American Cancer Society and the U. S. Public Health Service for this reason. This evidence has been mainly statistical, so far, which leaves it open to the charge of fallacious reasoning. Those physicians who are proponents of tobacco point out that the statisticians can show a very close correlation between the occurence of drownings and the consumption of ice cream cones—obviously not related to each other, but happening to occur in the same seasons.

They point out that the great majority of cigarette smokers do not die of lung cancer, and many non-smokers do. Nevertheless, sound statistical analysis has often suggested relationships, which upon further investigation proved true.

We do know that certain chemicals which have proved to produce cancer in animals are contained in small amounts and produced at certain temperatures in the burning of any hydrocarbon including tobacco, coal, oils and wood. We also know that the burning tip of a cigarette has a much higher temperature than that of a cigar or pipe, and that cigar or pipe smokers do not show an excess of lung cancer, though they do show a slight excess of cancer of the lip and mouth. Finally, a careful microscopic study of the finer branches of the bronchial tubes of heavy cigarette smokers has recently shown a thickening and overgrowth of the delicate cells which line these tiny tubes, which may or may not be a precursor of cancer.

Like the possible relationships between saturated fats in the diet and arteriosclerosis, we just don't know yet, for sure, but we'll find out in due time.

Circulatory Diseases

In addition to the suspected relationship between lung cancer and heavy cigarette smoking, there is pretty good evidence that these same excessive cigarette smokers succumb more frequently to diseases of the heart and circulatory system. There is no doubt that discontinuing cigarettes will relieve and often cure Buerger's Disease, a peculiar and not uncommon condition in which the extremities become cold and numb due to spasm of the arteries in the hands or feet or both.

So that's about the score against tobacco, especially cigarettes. Why does its use continue to increase? Well, let's look at some of the possible reasons.

Why Do We Smoke?

There is no doubt that many adults, some more than others, never quite get over their sucking instinct. In infancy, it brought them food, and in adults the lips remain one of the erotic stimulation areas. We see this among infants who suck their thumb or a pacifier, school children who suck their bubble gum or candy, and business men who suck their pencil, cigarette, pipe or cigar. Sucking is a basic instinct and in general no physiological harm comes of it.

How I used to envy, as a child, the bearded old janitor of our church. During the services he sat in a comfortable chair tipped back against a little recess, just in sight of our family pew, but out of sight of the pulpit and most of the congregation. There he relaxed sucking continuously on hard white peppermint candies. No sooner was one gone than he would rattle the little paper sack in his coat pocket and pop another into his mouth. He fairly made me drool, and he was much more fascinating than the sermon.

One day I bought a penny's worth of the very same white peppermints and saved them for church. When the sermon started I surreptitiously slipped one into my mouth. Hardly had I had the first good suck, however, when Mother held out her handkerchief for me to spit it into, and that was that.

At home she told me I mustn't chew gum or candy in church. I defended myself with the case of the janitor. She explained that he was an old man, didn't have much fun anyway and that his breath smelled better with peppermints than without. In retrospect, I think it had something to do with alcoholic halitosis.

So that's one reason people smoke tobacco.

Another is that it has somehow gained the reputation of being soothing, especially the pipe which is associated with relaxation and comfortable contemplation. Nicotine is officially listed as a narcotic, producing drowsiness and relaxing spasms. In large doses, or for those unaccustomed to it, it produces nausea and vomiting as many small boys learn to their sorrow. The effect of nicotine after it's burned and sucked in is not so certain.

Tobacco smoke, whatever it is, actually increases the pulse rate and tends to constrict the peripheral arteries, thus momentarily raising the blood pressure a little. Cigarette smokers are more apt to seek stimulation from their smoke. They say it overcomes drowsiness and they can think better. Anyway, it makes them feel different in some subtle way, and that's apparently what they seek. The same goes for chewing tobacco and using snuff. Thank goodness, a greater consciousness of sanitation and the high cost of cleaning spitoons seems to have limited this form of indulgence in recent years.

Another reason people—especially young people—smoke is that it gives them a feeling of daring, braggadocio and sophistication. It identifies them as part of "the gang." Others smoke, so they want to.

Tobacco is undoubtedly habit-forming, but not in the same way as opiates where a tolerance is built up, more are constantly required to produce the same sensations, and extremely painful withdrawal symptoms result when their use is discontinued.

Effects of Quitting

Withdrawal of tobacco does not produce serious symptoms—none, in fact—except those which might be expected from breaking any other motor habit. The former smoker doesn't know what to do with his hands and his sucking instinct; hence he gets nervous and may imagine great suffering, but he gets over it shortly. This is not to say it is easy to quit smoking. Some people say they can't, and many doctors let them continue rather than aggravate whatever else is the matter with them by this period of nervousness. But I have yet to see anything but good effects from stopping smoking. If the new abstainer is really upset by his nervousness, small amounts of tranquilizers for a while may see him through more comfortably.

A Bad Habit

The continuous use of tobacco is a bad habit. It is dirty, expensive, often annoys other people, burns holes in your clothes and stains your teeth. It is often harmful to the heart and circulation and it may trigger lung cancer. It does you no discernible good. It brands you as an infantile sucker or one who is so insecure he has to prove his security by doing what others do.

A Pleasant One

Yet, I dearly love my cigarettes. I try to keep them down to less than one package a day. The doctor says I should quit. That's easy, as Mark Twain said, "I've quit smoking dozens of times." But if anything really serious were the matter with me, I'd quit for good, and as Mr. Eisenhower said, "I'd never go through the 'agony' of quitting again."

Blessed Be the Permissive

That seems to be the attitude of most people who smoke. And I can only wish for them from the nonsmokers, the attitude of my dear wife. As she cleans the ash trays, airs out the apartment, and subtly lets me know how much it costs for an invisible patch on that last burn in my trousers, her attitude is—permissive.

Advertising and Youth

Because many executives have been concerned with the smoking of their children or grandchildren, there is one thing I would have the temerity to suggest to the cigarette purveyors: that their hard-sell advertising will someday turn on them. It is especially bad for the young who, in view of the medical facts available today, face a serious decision whether or not they wish to run the risk of cigarette-produced lung cancer, or an impaired circulatory system, or enslavement to a dirty and expensive habit. Instead of weighing the pros and cons, they are virtually hypnotized into concluding that the only way to be cool, sophisticated, grown-up, attractive to your girl- or boy-friend, be a real athlete and a man of affairs, is to smoke this or that kind of cigarette.

And there's nothing stronger than the feeble voice of the parents and school teachers to offset it. The public schools in many states are required to teach something about the evil effects of alcohol and tobacco. But how can they and parents compete with the effective extra-sensory perception techniques so skillfully used in these ads: the beautiful scenery, the beautiful girls and boys, the heroic appeal of athletes, the fetching jingles and impressive slogans? There was a time when the liquor salesmen used this method of advertising. How different are their still attractive but controlled ads today. The Eighteenth Amendment taught them what an aroused prohibitionist bloc can do.

Filter Facts

Finally, and incidentally, filters on cigarettes do little except cut down some of the throat-irritating elements of the smoke, or cut down the whole effluent so much that one gets no satisfaction and therefore smokes twice as many.

SLEEPING PILLS

Insomnia is a common complaint among executives. For some, it's almost inherent in their job. The executive's work is never completely finished, and whether he knows it or not, he carries his problems with him whether in the office, at home, on the golf course, or just fishing. Not that he necessarily worries about them or even mentions them, but they're there in the back of his mind, all the time. And this is not an unmixed blessing.

A Wakeful but Relaxed Mind

Often the solution of some of his most vexing problems will come to him in the middle of the night, or on the golf course, or while he's doing some recreational reading. This is because, when he's relaxed, away from the hurly-burly of the office, enjoying the pleasures of the outdoors or the comfort of his bed, his mind has time for more free association of long-forgotten experiences and the ideas derived from them. Suddenly a key word in casual conversation, or a familiar pleasing sight, or an odor, or a combination of these and other things, occurring while his mind is relaxed and receptive, will bring him the flash of what seems a new idea which may lead to the solution of a problem.

It is much the same process we all experience as we get older, inability to recall a certain word or a name. We say, "I'll think of it in a minute," and usually we do. The memory association paths in the brain are momentarily blocked by trying too hard to bring up the forgotten name. After a few moments relaxation of that particular pathway, the name comes to us out of a clear sky. So it is with some problems that seem insoluble. We bear down too heavily on them and block the delicate pathways of the mind. It's natural, and nothing to be worried about. In fact, worry makes it worse.

Not an Occupational Hazard

So I don't class insomnia as an occupational hazard among executives. It's seldom serious, and the main thing is not to get worried about it. It's best not to talk about it or get to complaining to your wife or anyone else. The more attention you pay to it, the worse it may get, and the sympathetic concern of others increases your own concern.

Rest Without Sleep

As a matter of fact, we all get plenty of sleep unless we're seriously ill or in great pain. Nature arranges this for us in quite a positive way. Observations in the military and in numerous scientific laboratories have shown that when fatigue is great enough, the necessity for sleep will overcome all other desires, even that of self-preservation in the face of danger. To be sure, we all seem to feel better when we can follow our accustomed pattern of eight to ten hours' good sleep every night. But to miss that for several nights, or even for quite a little while, is not serious, especially if we can rest lying down with our working clothes off for the accustomed number of hours. That in itself will relieve fatigue, both physically and mentally providing we don't stew about it. Read a good book, or do some writing with a lap-board, or just lie back and relax, count sheep if you will.

When Help is Needed

Nevertheless, as the good doctor on the night plane implied, there may come a time when unnatural conditions, or continuous unrelieved worry or other vicissitudes may call for a little help in the way of drugs—sleeping pills—and there's no reason for not using them under the restrictions imposed by the doctor, and with the precautions suggested here.

Ancient Uses and Hazards

Sleep-producing drugs have been known for centuries, probably starting with opium and its derivatives and cannabis or hemp derivatives or alcohol which was the commonest anesthetic before ether and chloroform. The "mickey finn," once accessible to conniving barkeepers, robbers and those who were paid to "shanghai" men for the navies and merchant vessels of the olden days, was once in common use. It was "knock-out drops" (chloral hydrate), and if the man was drunk enough he hardly noticed the bitter taste of a few drops in his last drink. It sometimes resulted, however, in death from overdosage, and the barkeeper didn't get his cut when a supposed drunk was put on board ship and turned out to be a corpse next morning. The opiates, too, carried a certain mortality, especially when combined with the shock of old-time surgery.

Tailor-Made to Fit

Today most of the sleeping pills are derivatives of the barbiturates, which, compared to the opium cup or the mickey finn are relatively harmless. There is a great variety of these derivatives, some with undesirable side-effects for some people such as headache or "hangover" next day, some quick-acting but of short duration so that there is early morning wakefulness, some slow-acting to produce continued sleep in the early morning, some little more effective than tranquilizers, discussed below, which are really a different class of drugs.

Your doctor will know which of these several choices is best for your particular needs and in what quantity. Unlike morphine or chloral hydrate, in both of which the difference between a therapeutic and fatal dose may be small, the barbiturates offer a wide margin of safety.

Let the Doctor Take Your Measure

So if you're really troubled about insomnia and it worries you more than it should, by all means see your doctor and tell him the whole story. The only way you can get a really effective sleeping pill is by prescription anyway. The doctor may have you try out two or three varieties before finding just the right one to meet your needs. Then remember what he tells you about its use.

Simple, Safe Precautions

You can easily become dependent upon sleeping pills and think you are unable to get to sleep without them. In this sense they may be habit forming, and it's a bad habit to get into. Often just having a pill handy at your bedside will assure you enough so that you will go to sleep without it. So don't take it unless you must.

If you need a pill, take it before midnight. Those who toss around until two or three in the morning and then take the pill are due for a "hangover" next morning which may last all day, or at least until noon. Your mind is not functioning at anywhere near its best when there's any remnant of the drug in your system.

Don't combine sleeping pills with alcohol. Perhaps a nightcap highball is all you need to get right to sleep. If so, don't take a pill. Or, if you go to bed under the influence of alcohol, don't take a pill. The barbiturates are much more potent when combined with alcohol, often too potent to be safe.

Don't leave the bottle of pills by the bedside. Instead, put out the prescribed dosage on your bedside table, then put the bottle back in the medicine chest. One of the characteristics of most sleeping pills is that they tend to destroy memory of recent events. So you may sleep awhile, then awaken and forget that you have already had the prescribed amount and proceed to take a second and even a third dose. I often wonder how many reputed suicides due to overdosage of sleeping pills were really people who went to bed inebriated, then proceeded to take one dose after another during the night because of simple forgetfulness.

Finally, stick a pin in the cork of the bottle, or stick a piece of scotch tape over it, so you won't mistake it for aspirin or something else when you go to the medicine cabinet in the dark—which, of course, you shouldn't do anyway. And be sure to keep all drugs, including aspirin, out of reach of children.

With these precautions and knowledge of their proper use, occasional resort to sleeping pills is often justified.

TRANQUILIZERS

Great strides have been made in recent years in research, mainly conducted or financed by the pharmaceutical industry, on a whole family of drugs for bringing greater tranquility to the troubled human mind. As a group these are mainly the so-called ataraxics which, roughly translated from the Greek, means "without anxiety." Most of them are derivatives of, or chemically related to, a remedy long known in southern Asia as a cathartic and a cure for intestinal worms. It came from the root of the plant called *Rauwolfia serpentinum*. From that crude and not too satisfactory worm cure in the hands of the pharmaceutical chemists have come this new group of drugs which, for the first time, are making it possible for many people to leave mental hospitals, allaying the unjustified fears and apprehensions which beset so many, soothing nerves and reducing blood pressure.

Numerous Varieties

In the annual edition of pharmaceutical specialties for the physician's ready reference, there are now over fifty remedies listed under this heading. There can be no doubt of their usefulness to the present-day physician. Fortunately, they are only available on prescription; otherwise, there are so many people nowadays with so many real or imagined anxieties that they would most surely be taken in harmful amounts and become habit forming for a great many. Some are fairly potent; others, milder. Some of the more potent have undesirable side-effects on some people and are used only as a calculated risk for the patient who is violently disturbed. Ten milligrams of one may be a toxic dose, while 1,000 milligrams a day of another may be an ordinary dose. When handled with skill and experience and under close medical supervision, they are a boon to that portion of mankind subject to nervous and mental disorders.

Numerous Uses

But here again, some people and perhaps especially executives, are sometimes subjected to a series of frustrations, continued anxieties, failures and tragedies, which are just too much for that particular individual to stand and remain healthy. Then is the time to see your doctor and let him know just how much pressure you are under. He may decide to help you with a mild tranquilizer of one kind or another, either temporarily or for some little time. He knows how to choose the one that will give you greater peace of mind without impairing your mental agility. Under these circumstances tranquilizers may be a great boon to you, and under these conditions I have never known them to do harm.

Self-Medication Dangers

I have known a few executives who ran into trouble with tranquilizers. Perhaps they were men who never should have been executives in the first place, or who never should have accepted the responsibilities involved in their last promotion. Perhaps they would have been all right if the market had remained stable, or that strike hadn't occurred, or that a competitor hadn't hit so hard. But these are the ups and downs of modern business which almost no one can foresee. They call for leaders with a steady hand, a keen mind and a strong spirit. Tranquilizers will not give them any of these if they don't have them already. All tranquilizers can do is tide them over some of the unbearably rough spots, when they're used properly under medical supervision.

Those who got into trouble took matters into their own hands and by fair means or foul got additional supplies of these potent medicines. Reasoning like my Uncle Peacey, who thought if a little of that medicine made him feel better, a whole lot more taken at once would cure him, they doubled and trebled the dose and went on what amounts to a prolonged tranquilizer binge. They did themselves no good, but neither the doctor nor the tranquilizer can be blamed.

To Be or Not to be Tranquil?

Let's face it. There are times in an executive's life when he can't and shouldn't, be tranquil. He's in the middle of a crisis and he's got to see it through. At the same time, he will impair his efficiency if he's overwrought. A good night's sleep will do him good, even if it does require a tranquilizer or a sleeping pill. The doctor is the one to help him with this, and he's foolish if he doesn't seek such help when he needs it.

STIMULANTS

Some people never need a stimulant. They're stimulated all the time anyway. They're what the psychiatrists call the "motor-manic type." With some of them, the problem is to get them to sit still long enough to do some serious thinking. Others, and this seems to include the great majority, do feel that they need a mild stimulant from time to time to overcome fatigue, ready them for extraordinary effort, or just to shake off the shackles of boredom. They most commonly resort to . . .

Coffee, Tea and Cocoa

As most people know, coffee contains a drug called caffeine. As a medicine it is used to stimulate the failing heart, to overcome the effects of narcosis such as that produced by alcohol, opiates or an overdose of sleeping pills. As a beverage in coffee, it is used to chase the last vestiges of sleep from the brain in the morning, or to keep awake when on night duty or when short of sleep, or just to make one feel more alert for the demands of the day's work. In the navy it is well-nigh a universal and continuous drink, as is the case in some offices.

The average cup of coffee made in the usual manner contains about five grains of caffeine, a minimal dose, much smaller than would be used therapeutically, and it does seem to "wake up" the mental processes. Without cream, milk or sugar it has virtually no calories, so does not add to our excess weight. I can't see that it does any harm to those who are not sensitive to it. It's a pleasant and relaxing custom to take a coffee break with friends, or to sip a cup with confreres at the desk or workbench.

A committee of the California Legislature in 1961 calculated that the state lost many millions of dollars yearly because of the coffee-break custom among state employees, and there was no evidence submitted to show that work neglected during that time was made up because of the stimulation of the caffeine.

As I write this, I look out on the East River where about fifty men are building a new parking garage and marina out over the water. Between 9:30 and 10 each morning one of the younger men walks three blocks to a restaurant and brings back a large carton with a pot of coffee, cream and sugar and paper cups and passes it around among the others wherever they are working. The temperature is just below freezing, with a strong northwest wind. I don't know, but my guess is that the men get more, rather than less done for that spot of warmth and of caffeine.

Except for those who are sensitive to coffee, little if any harm is done by it. Judging by the number of cups consumed daily by some people, I am sure there are those who are immune to the effects of caffeine.

Caffeine in Tea

What is not generally known is that there is likewise caffeine in tea, though usually in smaller amounts when made in the ordinary way, that is, by pouring boiling water on it, or dipping the tea bag into the boiling water. When made in the old English manner, however—heating the pot, using a generous pinch of black tea to the cup, pouring in the boiling water and letting it "steep" for five to ten minutes—I doubt if it contains much less caffeine per cup than coffee.

Tea also contains small amounts of tannic acid, considered a tonic for the stomach. Judging from the effects of a few small granules of tannic acid on the tongue, I have no doubt that it does tend to pucker up an otherwise flatulent stomach. It does little if any harm, except for those who have a stomach ulcer. Without cream or sugar it has no caloric value.

Caffeine's Cousin, Theobromin

Cocoa and most chocolate drinks contain another well known drug, theobromin, which has effects similar to caffeine, but somewhat weaker. Well diluted with milk it does little or no harm, though the number of calories is significant.

Various and Sundry Pills

Variously known as pep pills, goof pills, brain bombers and other sobriquets invented by the youthful slang of the day (and little understood by the "squares") these need not usually bother the business executive. Since he may hear them referred to in connection with school examinations or athletic contests, a word about them may not be amiss while we're talking about stimulants.

A few years ago it was discovered that amphetamine, better known as benzidrine, mixed with aromatic oils and packed in a nasal inhaler with cotton, would give quick relief to the stuffy nose caused by colds when sucked in through the nostrils, first one, then the other. Since this stuffiness is caused by a swelling of the membranes lining the nostrils, and this in turn often blocks the natural drainage of the numerous nasal sinuses, its temporary relief often restores that drainage and therefore relieves the headaches so common with a cold in the head. There is no doubt that it and several similar derivatives are helpful for some people's colds when used early.

The effect does not last long, and the use of the inhaler must be repeated frequently, but it is sometimes enough to tide over the early symptoms of a cold and avoid the spread of this infection to the sinuses and the lower respiratory system.

Sniffers, not Cribbers

Repeated users discovered, however, that it also gave the brain some stimulation, a feeling of elation and the illusion that they could think more quickly. Thus it was noted that the sale of these inhalers increased during the examination time, and some students were found using the inhaler throughout the writing of their exams. Later after the inmates of one of the largest prisons went on an unexplainable riotous binge, it was found that they had been saving inhalers dispensed in the infirmary, soaking the cotton contents in water and drinking the solution. After being quieted, they were generally unable to sleep.

Inherent Dangers

Most of the "pep pills" are derivatives of this family of chemicals. They have a legitimate use in medicine in treating overdosage of opiates or sleeping pills and in treating diseases and injuries of the brain which cause undue sleepiness. But they must be used with caution, since they do increase the pulse rate, the blood pressure, and cause constriction of the coronary and other arteries. Hence they may precipitate a heart attack in older people. Even among the young, they are not drugs to be used indiscriminately. Like most drugs of this kind, when the effect is over, a reaction sets in, and the nose, or the cerebral arteries, or whatever has been most affected, are stuffier than they were before.

OPIUM DERIVATIVES AND MARIJUANA

These might have been discussed under sedatives, but they are a group which will seldom bother the executive except as they may account for the strange behavior of an occasional employee who was an addict and denied it before he was employed, or who, for the many bizarre reasons which try to explain addictions, has become one. They can be dealt with very briefly here.

There are many derivatives of opium which have been a great blessing to mankind. They include morphine, codeine, heroin and others, but not cocaine, which is obtained from coca leaves, or marijuana, which comes from a species of hemp.

Underground Addicts

In many parts of the world there are no restrictions on the sale of opium. It is cheap and is used by a considerable portion of the population who smoke it in a long pipe. If used in moderation, it induces relaxation and pleasant dreams and makes an otherwise hard life more tolerable.

In this country, the Harrison Anti-Narcotic Act places severe restrictions on the dispensing of any drug derived from opium or containing such derivatives, and any cocaine or its derivatives. Thus the addicts have been driven underground and must pay exorbitant prices for inferior products which are smuggled in. Although once they are apprehended they may be treated free by the Public Health Service and practically all of them freed of the addiction, a discouraging number revert as soon as discharged. They constitute a very difficult medical problem, much more difficult than alcoholism, but fortunately not so extensive. The drug is self-administered with the hypodermic needle. When the addict is in short supply he will go to almost any lengths from robbery to murder to obtain what he needs.

"Snow"

Much the same things are true of the cocaine addict except that he may snuff the powder into his nose or administer a water-solution with a nose dropper.

"Reefers"

Marijuana, also spelled mariahuana, is a derivative of one of the hemp species. It was formerly smuggled in largely from Mexico, but it is a sturdy plant, somewhat resembling giant ragweed and about as wide-spread and prolific. It has been found growing in vacant lots, in New York's Central Park, in flower gardens and in one case a prison yard. The dried leaves are smoked as cigarettes called "reefers" and produce a form of inebriation characterized by loss of inhibitions, loss of time sense but not of rhythm and mental exaltation. An employee under its influence may seem to be drunk but is without the alcoholic breath. He may be dangerous and is certainly untrustworthy, so must be dealt with promptly and firmly. The addiction is not severe, being easier to break than alcoholism. If he values his job, the medical department working with Personnel may often save him.

CHAPTER

8

MAKING THE BEST OF WHAT WE HAVE

OFF TO A GOOD START

WITH few exceptions, we are all born with many rich endowments. We have the power of locomotion and speech, sight, hearing and the other special senses, a brain superior to that of any other living thing on earth, which enables us to think, remember, reason, communicate, record and invent. Naturally, some of us are born with greater gifts than others. If we all had equal or similar gifts, *everyone* might be an executive.

One of the most important things in life is to make the very best of our remarkable gifts. This means doing all we can to develop and enhance those special abilities with which a kind Providence provided us. Of equal importance is overcoming in one way or another deficiencies with which we were born, or which we may acquire, so that they will interfere least with what we really want to do.

THE RACE IS NOT ALWAYS TO THE SWIFT

Unfortunately, but inevitably, we will not all withstand life's vicissitudes equally well. The inexorable attritions of daily life will dull or destroy some of our most precious God-given and self-developed abilities. Almost no one escapes entirely, so it's wise to be somewhat prepared for them. In addition, therefore, to making the best of our inborn gifts, it is of the utmost importance to make the best of what is left us when accident, illness or just plain wear and tear leaves us with certain mental or physical impairments. Some of these are more serious than others. Many are not serious at all, except as we make them so by self-pity, lack of courage or just plain fear born of ignorance. With determination, much can be done to overcome even the more serious handicaps, either by adjustment, retraining or change of pace or goal. The modern executive must have made the best of at least some of his inborn abilities or he would not be where he is. But he may not be prepared to meet the handicaps that befall so many. This chapter should help prepare him.

TURNED DOWN FOR LIFE INSURANCE?

One of the first "setbacks," and often one of the least serious, comes when the young executive decides he needs more life insurance and his application is declined or "rated up" as a result of his physical examination. This is frequently his first inkling that he is not a perfect physical specimen. He may indignantly decline the higher priced policy which is offered, appealing to his personal doctor to show the company that they are wrong. Or he may accept the higher rating reluctantly and go into a blue funk over the fact that he is not immortal. Both the protest and the blue funk are quite unnecessary. Let's see why.

Just remember, it's not the company medical examiner who rates you up. It's those medical underwriters back in the home office. There isn't much your doctor can do about it. These underwriters are, on the whole, a skilled group of experts. They know far better than your physician which category of risks you belong in, because they know beyond a doubt the mortality rate to be expected among many thousands of people just your age, height, weight and body-build with exactly the same impairments you have; perhaps a slight rise in blood pressure combined with a little overweight, persistent acceleration of the pulse-rate and maybe a slight bit of albumin in the urine.

WHAT ACTUATES THE ACTUARIES

They *know,* as a result of the periodic medico-actuarial analysis of their claim-rate, that a hundred thousand such individuals will, *as a group,* have a death-rate higher than a similar group without these impairments; they know exactly how much greater that death-rate will be, and how much extra they must charge *the group* to make up for the increased risk. The whole thing is based on averages, and they know what they must do to keep the insuring company solvent. You certainly wouldn't want to be insured with a company whose insolvency in years to come would make it impossible to pay your full claim.

NO ONE IS AVERAGE

Of course, there is no such thing as an average *individual.* Averages apply only to groups. Your own doctor knows you as an individual, and you can depend on his advice as it fits you personally. He may decide that the whole thing is a tempest in a teapot as far as *you* are concerned and you need pay no attention to it. Or he may look upon this as an early warning that you are veering off onto the wrong track physically and advise you to reduce your weight. This, in itself, may lower your blood pressure, calm down your pulse and eliminate the trace of albumin. If this is necessary, right now is the best time to find it out and do something about it. Then, a year from now, you may pass the insurance examination with flying colors. But don't refuse the policy. The company will adjust the premium back to normal rates if your slight impairments are cleared up next year. If they don't clear up, or by any chance get worse, the premium can't be increased, and you are lucky to have the coverage for your family.

MAKING THE BEST OF WHAT WE HAVE NOW

In the life and health insurance business we see so many tragedies of hardship due to some young executive failing to make realistic plans for the future, that we seem justified in emphasizing this important means of making the best of what we have. It is not pleasant, I know, to dwell on the possibilities of death or disablement. But the good executive must learn to think of all possible future exigencies which might affect his business. And like everyone else, he cannot, in all conscience, do less than make sensible provision for those he loves most.

To cite just one typical case (and I could cite thousands): A young executive of my acquaintance was going great guns—president of his small but prosperous one-man business, a distinguished military record, membership in the best clubs, popular, living graciously but expensively, giving his little family "all the advantages." Suddenly, he died of a heart attack at the age of forty-eight. Evidently this was the last thing he ever thought of or planned for.

His estate provided just enough for his son to finish college, and his widow to take a small apartment while she recovered her emotional equilibrium sufficiently to look for a job. She had beauty, charm and intelligence, but she had never worked in her life and had been reared in the lap of luxury.

Discouraging years have followed. Turned down on job after job, those she did get proved unsuitable and she resigned or was let out. At the moment, she stands in line each week with the other unemployed of her neighborhood, reporting that she has been unable to find a job that week, drawing her meager unemployment compensation, and hoping something turns up before it runs out.

Her brilliant, successful and relatively well-to-do husband could easily have afforded a substantial life insurance policy, but didn't think he needed it—yet.

WE ARE NEITHER IMMORTAL NOR INDESTRUCTIBLE

Let's face it. None of us is immortal. Many people do die before they are fifty—more than most of us realize.

Nor are we by any means indestructible. I have seen many men and women utterly shattered by an injury or illness which leaves them with some permanent handicap. Even this unpleasant subject deserves a little discussion here. As I know from experience and observation, the executive who plans his future to include the possibility (however remote) of disablement is better prepared if something does happen than one who acts as if he were immortal or indestructible.

In general, executives have a great deal of willpower. Come hell or high water, they do whatever they set out to do. This is all in their favor when illness or accident does strike, and I have seen many of them stage a comeback that would be impossible for less determined individuals.

I think of one man, for instance, a brilliant student in college, endowed with a remarkable mind and a charming personality who was forging ahead in his chosen field and looked like one of the nation's coming leaders in a few more years. Through no fault of his, his car turned over and burned. His life was saved, but his face was mutilated. Year after year for five years, the plastic surgeons worked on him, reconstructing nose, eyelids and ears, grafting skin little by little. When not in the hospital he stayed indoors at home because people on the street shuddered when they looked at him. Today, his face is not only presentable but pleasant looking. The skin is not very flexible, but there shines from his eyes a spirit of determination, mixed with compassion and understanding such as few ever attain on this earth. He lost five years, but today he's at the very top of his profession, and a better loved man you never saw. Don't think he didn't have his days of despair, but he went right on doing what he was determined to do. One could well say that he gained from his misfortune. The two Presidents Roosevelt are other good examples of what determination will do.

On the other hand, some people are so completely demoralized after a crippling body blow that they never do succeed in patching their lives together again.

I knew another young executive, well on his way up in a technical field in which he had showed great promise in college. He really was a near genius in his line and was being admired and quoted by his colleagues all over the country. He contracted a virulent form of pulmonary tuberculosis. This was before we had the present wonder-drugs, and the only chance of saving him was rest in bed in a sanatorium, which might take several years. He was extremely resentful over his ill fate and resisted treatment at every turn. He would not stay in bed, said he couldn't quit smoking cigarettes, had to have the nurse take his temperature or he would put the thermometer on the table instead of in his mouth. He kept saying he had to get home and take care of his work and his family and why didn't we hurry up and cure him. The minute he recovered from a hemorrhage and got to feeling stronger, he'd go AWOL and visit his home for a few days. We pleaded with him, pointing out the risk he was taking, not only for himself but in spreading the infection to his family. He finally "signed out" without medical permission, went home, kept having repeated hemorrhages and died within the year. He was a brilliant engineer, but he had no brilliance or even good judgment once he was disabled.

LIGHTNING DOES STRIKE

So, the first point I want to make here, especially for the younger executive on the way up, is that none of us is infallible, invincible or immortal. Disaster does strike a certain number. It usually comes suddenly and without warning. The wise young man on his way to being a top executive will give as much thought to assuring his own and his family's future security as he does to his business progress. This holds true no matter how hard he may be struggling to pay for a new home, make further investments in his business, or how attractive the stock market may look. Many a young man's rise to fame and glory has come about through a series of hairbreadth escapes and just plain luck. In the practice of medicine and in the insurance business, we see altogether too many of the unlucky ones. And who can say on whose shoulder Lady Luck will or will not ride?

Life insurance in *adequate* amounts and some kind of comprehensive health insurance for himself and family are among the first necessities in planning for the future. Family and creditors can be protected from the economic disaster of untimely death by adequate life insurance. The financial disaster of serious illness or accident can be largely averted by adequate health insurance.

HAVE A LOOK AT THE HANDICAPPED

One of the best ways to face reality is to give a little thought to it, and observe what happens to others who are physically handicapped. This has a direct bearing on employment of the handicapped worker, too, with which every executive should help. I know all about the workmen's compensation and disability insurance angle and it's not the bugaboo it's often made out to be.

I wish every executive who has anything to do with employment could make at least one visit to one of the rehabilitation centers scattered over the country. There he could see the amazing advances that have been made in this field of medicine, largely since the war. With the help of trained vocational counselors, occupational therapists, physiotherapists, ingenious makers of braces and other prosthetic devices, speech therapists, teachers of lip reading, and above all good nurses and doctors in the various specialities, some well-nigh incredible things happen to the physically handicapped to restore them to some kind of self-respecting usefulness.

A housewife with a back broken in such a way as to sever the spinal cord, who therefore is permanently paralyzed from the waist down, is taught to help herself to and from wheel-chair and bed, and to go about her household duties in a specially built kitchen with everything reachable from the chair.

A good chef who lost both legs in an elevator accident learns to get around on two artificial limbs, but he can no longer be safe around the ranges, so he sits on a stool and acts as a checker in the kitchen where he can still plan menus and supervise his favorite dishes.

A brilliant lawyer paralyzed in both arms from polio still has slight movement in some fingers of each hand. By getting him a special electric-touch typewriter, he is able to carry on his business with his partners.

An expert mechanic who will never be able to use his hands or arms again has become quite famous and makes a good living painting pictures with the brushes held in his teeth.

An elderly doctor who suffered a stroke which affected one arm, one leg and his speech, is given passive massage and carefully graduated exercises as well as speech therapy each day until he's almost as good as new and can carry on his teaching and writing duties.

Of course, there is a limit to what can be done for those who lack the determination, or those too badly handicapped to have much left for salvage. But it's the spirit that counts, and even those who have just a little determination can have it enormously enhanced by encouragement, constructive treatment and empathy (not sympathy).

JUST ONE BREAK

When a handicapped individual has been successfully rehabilitated, he has already shown extraordinary courage, but he needs much more. The greatest of all discouragements comes when he tries to find a job. The majority of employers will have nothing to do with the handicapped. This is in spite of the fact that the records compiled by the organization called "JOB" (Just One Break) show that as a group the trained handicapped person has far better motivation toward his work than the average worker. His attendance record surpasses the average, and when properly placed in a job he can handle, his output often is so great as to embarrass his fellows.

Once an employer accepts a member of the JOB organization, he is assured that if for any reason the individual turns out to be unsatisfactory, he need only let the organization know and it will save him the embarrassment of discharging the worker. They take their member off his hands, help analyze the reasons for failure, and proceed to try to find another employer.

SOME HAPPY ADJUSTMENTS

It is always a joy to me, and it should be to the employer, to see a handicapped individual well placed in employment. I have mentioned the chef-amputee who is happy and valuable on a stool as a checker in the kitchen, also the lawyer with the electric-touch typewriter.

One Sunday I went over to get a photograph of the old William H. Park Laboratory on New York's East River before it was to be torn down. There was no one in sight on the grounds and the gate was open. As I strolled in toward the building an uncanny, sepulchural voice seemed to come out of the sky.

"Are you looking for someone?" it said.

It so startled me that I wondered for a moment if it could be the voice of dear old Dr. Park himself from beyond the pearly gates.

Looking around, I found a tall elderly man standing outside the watchman's shack, holding a wire-connected gadget to the front of his neck. I introduced myself and told him my errand. Through the tube, which I then saw was connected to a loud speaker atop his shack, he replied in the same sepulchral tone that I was most welcome, to go on with the photo and let him know when I came out.

It turned out that he was a long-time city employee whose larynx had been removed on account of cancer some years ago. He could speak only with the help of this sounding tube, which had been connected to the loud-speaker so that his low artificial voice could be heard all over the grounds. He showed me the other wire that he plugged into the telephone when it rang or he needed instructions or help.

He was proud of himself and his ability to earn a good living and maintain his civil service status. Later I learned from the Department of Health that he was the most dependable watchman they had ever had.

What a happy placement of a man who might well have gone into the discard, perhaps at best ended up on the relief rolls!

Speaking of voice handicaps, I recall an intelligent middle aged woman who came in for placement one day. She had suffered from a tumor of one of the endocrine glands, which though removed, had left her with a deep bass voice and a beard, due to hormone imbalance. Her appearance was good, thanks to regular shaving and cosmetics, but her voice was really startling. For years she had been a highly successful department head in a large store, but this involved much contact with customers.

She explained that when her voice changed so markedly, it proved a handicap, especially with the public. The store was undergoing a recession and had nothing else for her.

It so happened that the local large air terminal was looking for an announcer on the public address system, a well-paid job requiring high intelligence, quick thinking and a good voice. She got the job and is doing marvelously at it. Her voice is perfectly clear throughout the terminal. It has the pleasant lilt of a female voice and the clear carrying qualities of a male voice. She never meets the public, and her fellow workers appreciate her personality, sense of humor and dependability.

WHAT DOES THE JOB REALLY REQUIRE?

Bert Hanman, long-time consultant for the Veterans Hospitals in Boston, and his colleagues, were among the first in this country to try to analyze the exact physical requirements of each job in the Kaiser shipbuilding industries during the war, when labor was scarce. The medical department was furnished with an index showing, for each job category, how much time the workers spent on their feet, indoors or outdoors, climbing ladders or stairs, lifting heavy or light articles, importance of vision and hearing, manual dexterity, and so forth.

As applicants with physical impairments were examined, the doctor could check off the things he could not do. For example, a man with an arthritic spine might not be able to do a job which required considerable stooping, bending or lifting, but he could do everything else that might be required; a man with a heart condition might be unable to do any job that required much physical exertion, but could do bench or office work; a man with an artificial leg might be good for any job that did not require climbing or work on a scaffold. In this way, they were able to tap that great reservoir of handicapped people, most of whom were eager to find jobs and determined to make good.

The Company's experience with the group was most favorable, once the leadermen and foremen became accustomed to observing the restrictions under which the individual was to work. I don't suppose the percentage of handicapped so employed came to five per cent of the total employees, but in an enterprise of this size, it means jobs for a very great number who had been unemployed for many years.

In later studies of the Swedish shipbuilding practices where this man-job-matching process had been followed longer, there is a report of an applicant who had one artificial leg, a stiff elbow from an old fracture, was blind in one eye and hard of hearing. It turned out that he was capable of doing nearly eighty per cent of the jobs in the yard, and when hired did very well.

A CREATIVE PERSONNEL POLICY

In this country the understandable but often unrealistic desire of employers to select only those applicants who are paragons mentally and physically, has led to unanticipated abuses of our system of unemployment benefits. There is nothing that will make a man feel worthless more quickly than to be told repeatedly that his impairments disqualify him for a job. In this and other ways we create our own unemployables. I sometimes think their number is increasing every day. Every executive owes it to the society in which he has been so favored, to be a good citizen in that society and to create the image of his industry as a good citizen too.

One of the best ways to do this is to construct a personnel policy which will *try* at least to find a place for a reasonable number of the handicapped, even some of those whose only handicap is plain stupidity. It seems to me far better for industry to shoulder a fair share of responsibility for these people than to have them carried indefinitely on the relief rolls. Like the problem of alcoholism, it can be done if the chief executives of a business let it be known that they want it done. It has to come from the top. Once this is established, it is surprising how much humanitarian interest in the cause of helping the handicapped will be taken by supervisory personnel at all levels.

In one large organization that I know, there are eighteen or twenty epileptics. Most of them are under good control with modern medication, but occasionally one will have a seizure while at work. Twenty years ago in this organization an employee "having a fit" would disrupt the whole section for the rest of the day. Now, because of the humanitarian attitudes of the chief executives, the supervisors have learned to be kindly and patient with these unfortunates. They simply call the medical division, which responds promptly and wheels the victim away to the rest rooms. Fellow-workers are calm and sympathetic and do the best they can to keep up the output of the section despite the shortage of one person.

In this same organization a man who is totally blind, but whose eyes appear normal, sits behind a desk and listens to employees who have complaints. He has an engaging personality, a good sense of humor and a marvelous sense of human values. He listens carefully, deducing a great deal from the choice of words and tone of voice. If the complaint is justified, he reassures the individual that it will be remedied and sees that it is. If, as is most often the case, the individual is just blowing off steam and really has little to kick about, he then discloses his own blindness, always a surprise to his confrere, and says, "Well, things might be worse, hey?"

THE BUILT-IN SUCCESS MECHANISM

In thinking of those recently handicapped by injury or illness, including mental illness or "nervous breakdown," we tend to overlook the marvelous therapeutic effects of work. Most people—I won't say all—really have a pretty strong desire to do something useful and to earn a living. When this is denied them, even temporarily, they begin to disintegrate. We are all familiar with the "compensation neurosis" case, who, injured at work, remains incapacitated far longer than the injury alone seems to justify, and who is back at work, cured, shortly after he collects the award to which he and his lawyer think he is entitled.

Every individual has a "built-in success mechanism," some more than others. His natural tendency is to recover and get to some productive occupation, even when his injury or illness has been most grievous. But this mechanism is easily interfered with by the various tricks of the forebrain, by unconscious fears, by frustrations and sometimes by misdirected ambitions. Most often the harm is done by the unwitting suggestions of his friends and advisors, including his lawyer and sometimes his doctor.

This "built-in success mechanism" is a fascinating subject, well worth some study by any executive. A book entitled *Psycho-Cybernetics* by Maxwell Maltz (Prentice-Hall, Englewood Cliffs, N.J., 1960) discusses this in relatively plain terms, despite a title which might be discouraging to the busy executive. Dr. Maltz is a distinguished plastic surgeon with a remarkable insight into human psychology. He likens the human subconscious and nervous system to the electronic brain, which turns out the right answer only when the proper data is fed into it. Those who feed into their subconscious nothing but fear, discouragement, inferiority and expectations of failure, automatically condition their nervous system to produce failure. Those who feed into their subconscious nothing but courage, reassurance and determined expectations of success, will have success. These latter are the ones who usually recover most completely from any disability.

The "built-in success mechanism" is one of the most precious endowments with which we are born. It works all the time, even when we sleep. It is completely ruined, however, and never fully repaired, when the individual with any handicap whatsoever is repeatedly told that he's useless. Many employment offices do this unwittingly.

What has been said in this section is obviously largely in the hope of arousing the executive's thoughtful consideration of the handicapped in relation to his employment policies. There is a vast literature on this subject for the benefit of those who want specific, practical suggestions. It can be obtained from The President's Committee on Employment of the Handicapped, Washington 25, D.C.; the National Association of Manufacturers, New York, N.Y.; the Chamber of Commerce of the U.S., Washington, D.C.; and the

Association for the Aid of Crippled Children, 345 East 46 Street, New York, N.Y.

MAKING THE BEST OF WHAT WE HAVE (LEFT?)

Now to come back to making the best of what we have, despite the wear and tear of the years and the fortuitous illnesses and injuries which may beset any of us, we might entitle this last portion of the chapter "Making the Best of What We Have Left."

Most of us will lose some or all of our teeth and become accustomed to dental aides of one kind or another. Most of us will gradually develop impaired vision and become adjusted to various kinds of eyeglasses. Many of us will be forced to become inured to the jokes about baldness, or resort to a toupee. All of us will slow down, sooner or later, as we get older. We'll have to adjust to nine holes of golf instead of eighteen, to riding more and walking less. We may take comfort in the belief that our judgment gets better as our experience accumulates, and up to a point, there is some justification in this.

DELAYED ONSET OF EXECUTIVITIS

A few executives, and I think fewer than formerly, tend to become irascible as they get older. They seem to adopt the attitude that they have had more experience than anyone else in the business, that they haven't many years left and they'd better speak their mind now before it's too late. Others of these few seem to like to rest more and more on their laurels and to demand more and more obeisance from their underlings. In truth, they are so powerful in their business that sweet reasonableness seems to desert them, and they become the authoritarian monarchs of all they survey, respected for what they have done rather than what they are doing, but automatically surrounded by sycophants, and therefore feared.

Delayed cases of executivitis, I'd call them. It's too bad they hung on so long that they finally succumbed to it. These are sad cases, indeed, both from the medical and the business standpoint.

This affliction is like "halitosis"—their best friends won't tell them. They don't dare to.

EARLY RETIREMENT HAS VIRTUES

Personally, I am a strong believer in early retirement. Many will disagree with this opinion, mainly because they don't understand what I mean by retirement. Above all, I do not mean idleness. I think a man can and should be just as active mentally, even if not physically, after retirement as before. For a person with a really good executive's mind, this should pose no problem. By the very nature of this puzzling but enjoyable, fearful but intriguing, frustrating but satisfying, aloof but friendly, stodgy but fast-moving world we live in, he must, perforce, have developed over the years many absorbing interests outside his business. This is especially so if he makes a conscious effort to cultivate and participate in these interests throughout his active business career.

If, in addition, he has foreseen that no matter how generous his pension may seem when he's thirty-five, it will never provide for all the things he'd like to have and do after sixty-five, and has, therefore, managed some savings; and if he and his wife have faced the fact that they will have less to live on after retirement and have figured out together some of the more expensive things they can cheerfully do without, then truly retirement from an active business career can be a glorious "graduation" to freedom, joys of active accomplishment, and unhampered participation in many interesting fields of activity.

"EXIT SMILING"—AND EARLY

Every executive develops some sort of a technique to get rid of people who have stayed at his desk talking too long. But what a pest that sort of a person is. An executive often sizes up his subordinates by the time and manner of their exit. The one who states his business quickly, answers questions directly, gets his instructions clearly and then gets out quickly is the one to tie to.

How many, many people there are who don't know when they're through! Some executives are that way. They're really through, but won't admit it. They hang on for self-glorification, or inflated ego, or often because they don't know what else to do. Meanwhile, though they'd be the last to admit it, they're holding back younger often abler men. They stick to old procedures and principles which the business has outgrown, as everyone else knows. Finally they wind up an otherwise brilliant career, heartily disliked by everyone but misled by the few remaining sycophants who surround them.

Don't do it. Quit early rather than late. If you've selected and trained your subordinates right, they can run the business at least as well as you, and often better, although it may be hard for you to admit it. Once out of the office, stay out and let them alone. *Exit Smiling* was the title of the immortal Irvin S. Cobb's autobiography and last book. To that excellent motto, I just add—"And Early."

SOME EXCEPTIONS

There are a few exceptions to this rule, but they are fewer than most older executives like to think. The average age of our U.S. Senators always surprises me. There can be no doubt about the continued value and exceptional abilities of many of those who are well past seventy. They are some of the exceptions. Among others are Winston Churchill, Herbert Lehman and Charles de Gaulle. Over thirty years ago de Gaulle said, "The man of character finds an especial attractiveness in difficulty, since it is only by coming to grips with difficulty that he can realize his potentialities." And here he is at eighty still coming to grips with difficulty. Perhaps it is something like this that accounts for the exceptions. An outstanding exception is the "grand old man" to whom this book is dedicated.

SEX BECALMED

Besides hair, teeth, vision, hearing and athletic prowess, there is another loss that eventually comes to all as they grow older. When it does, it sometimes causes undue concern. Like loss of teeth, to some it happens fairly early, between forty and fifty. To others, quite late, perhaps seventy to eighty. It is the diminishing ability to perform sexually.

The concern aroused by this natural event is often unduly severe for both men and women, but especially for men. It can, and has become a neurosis in some cases. Magnified, this concern not infrequently leads to some rash behavior when, as people say, the man is old enough to know better. Let's have a look at it before concluding this chapter.

What I have to present here are my own conclusions based on extensive but conflicting medical and psychiatric literature, the experiences, trials and tribulations of some of my private patients, experiences as admissions officer in veneral disease clinics, and the strange mixture of fact, superstition and folklore gathered around army campfires. Many will disagree with my conclusions, but it seems to me that this is a sensible and generally factual presentation.

FAULTY FOLKLORE

Some boys grow into manhood with the idea that the regular and periodic emission of seminal fluid is as necessary to health as emptying the bladder or moving the bowels. Many have grown up with the belief that masturbation is harmful. Therefore, they feel they must have recourse to what they consider "normal" sex relations periodically or their health will suffer.

Neither of these ideas could be farther from the truth. Production of the sperm cell and the ovum may be likened to the blossom of the plant. In fact, this blossom might be called the sexual apparatus of the plant.

Under proper conditions of nurture such as just the right amount of sunshine, moisture and food, and in the absence of injury by parasites, the plant will come to maturity and produce blossoms indefinitely until it finally becomes too old. Then the blossoms disappear, but the plant lives on for quite some time. Or, when conditions are not just right, the plant stops blooming. It appears perfectly healthy, but just won't bloom. When the right conditions of environment are restored, it blooms again as beautifully as ever. With many plants, sweet peas for example, the more the blossoms are cut, the more the plant produces.

MADE TO ORDER

So it is with the human male. The more sperm used, the more produced during the active sexual life of the individual. But, as with the sweet pea, no harm is done by not using them at all. Through a delicate mechanism of adjustment, fewer are produced. No bladder will be ruptured; no bowel will be overdistended. When conditions are right again, as in a happy marriage, sexual activity will gradually develop and increase until a nice balance, pleasing to both partners is reached and maintained. With some it may continue well into the seventh decade. With others, it begins to decrease gradually as early as the fourth decade. Physically it need cause no concern.

Mentally, it may cause psychological problems, especially for men who do not understand it.

I once had a patient, a dear old man born of Italian peasant stock, who had prospered in this country and with his sweet little wife had brought forth a fine family including a lawyer, a doctor, and an artist. At the age of eighty-five he was clearing some fallen trees from his yard and developed a massive hernia or rupture. It was so large and so intractable to any other method of treatment that it called for surgical repair, the sooner the better.

His physician son, a good surgeon, and I pleaded with him to have it done, lest it become strangulated some day and threaten his life. But he would have none of surgery. He said he was afraid that "going under the knife" would destroy his sexual powers. And his wife, about his age, was as adamant as he.

A POWERFUL INSTINCT

Among the deepest instincts born in the male is that of procreation. In nearly every species (though not all) he is the aggressor. Upon this instinct and this aggression depend the survival of the species. Hence, it is understandable that most men become greatly concerned when they find their sexual powers diminishing. A few are impelled to strange and often dangerous extremes. They feel that they have to prove their continued virility to themselves by extra-marital relations which may be neither discreet nor safe, and which can lead to serious consequences ranging from veneral disease to blackmail. The risks they take are at such variance with their previous behavior that their doctor may wonder whether they are mentally unbalanced.

THE BEST OF ALL IS YET TO COME

The sunset years of life should be years of peace and tranquility. The heat of the noonday sexual urge is waning as it should and the cool of the afternoon and twilight is ours to anticipate and enjoy. There is no less affection between man and wife, but rather an even greater devotion to each other, a devotion which is born of the understanding that comes with the years together, the memory of the earlier problems of business and family, the fears and the joys shared together. They can finally become peacefully reconciled to each other's shortcomings. They can appreciate more fully than ever before the sterling good qualities of each partner. The good that is in all of us grows with the years and it sometimes takes years to learn to fully appreciate it. These years, beginning around the sixth decade, should be the richest, most peaceful and most enjoyable of all.

CHAPTER 9

THE WOMAN EXECUTIVE

Now the time has come to confess that what has been written thus far has had a pretty strong bias toward the male sex. This was done deliberately because of the preponderance of male business executives. But, while they may have a majority, they by no means have a monopoly in the executive field. History abounds in records of outstanding women such as Hatshepsut in the eighteenth Egyptian Dynasty through Cleopatra, Queen Victoria, Florence Nightingale, to our own era of outstanding business women such as Lord & Taylor's Dorothy Shaver and others. There is some evidence that the number of women occupying positions of high respect and authority in this country is growing. And well it should, as men continue to overcome their former irrational prejudice against female participation in business and politics.

UNCROWNED QUEENS OF BUSINESS

Besides the women recognized as executives now and in the past, there are the large number of women who may not have an executive title but who exercise important executive functions in business, industry and politics. They range all the way from wives to secretaries, supervisors, section-heads, bookkeepers and accountants. Just imagine, if you can, where their high-executive boss would be without them. Whether overt or subtle, the influence they bring to bear on husband or boss is sometimes considerable—literally startling in some cases.

I felt that way one time when I was enjoying a running correspondence with a U.S. Senator. It was partly humorous and partly serious, and was aimed at remedying some shortcomings in the public health law. His secretary evidently decided that since I was neither a constituent nor a large contributor to the Party, I needn't bother the Senator any more. His replies stopped. Two years later, when we met again socially, he asked why I had stopped writing him.

The uncrowned queens of business appear to exert their influence in a number of ways, some open and direct, others so subtle that they deserve passing mention.

Most frequently their executive functions develop through sheer ability. These women are intelligent, educated and skilled in their job. In addition to ability, they have the added advantage of feminine intuition. Granted that intuition may often be wrong, and that it cannot always be supported by logic, it's right often enough for men to be foolish not to take it into consideration at times.

Some women in business exert their influence through authority that has been delegated to them. I see many executives who are pretty stingy about openly delegating authority to obviously able women. They're pretty stingy about promotion, title and salary too. That's a hangover from the many cultures which relegate women to an inferior position.

Other women gain power in business by infiltration. Of course, men use this method too, but it is usually less subtle and more easily identified. With women, it is often associated with the so-called maternal instinct; the male boss is "her boy." He needs protection; he needs the woman's touch to do things for him—things that no one else is thoughtful or considerate enough to do. So far so good—and what a great help these thoughtful girls can be. No wonder we often say we couldn't do without them.

THE STRUGGLE FOR STATUS

This infiltration technique is often associated also with that green-eyed struggle for status. The idea seems to be "my boss is bigger than your boss; therefore, I'm bigger than you." Talk about men status-seekers—some women are the real experts at this game.

Did you ever, for instance, overhear a couple of secretaries jockeying for position to see who can put her boss on the phone last? If one can get the caller on the phone first and then let him wait a moment before announcing him, it seems to prove that her boss is bigger than the caller; hence, she is also bigger and smarter than the other secretary.

Of course, some of this is all right, but it can be carried too far almost before you know it, so that a secretary becomes the office bully.

Some women gain executive authority in business by usurpation. This is commonest when the boss is either lazy or indifferent, or when he is so harrassed by multiple problems that he is glad to have someone at hand who will take over some responsibilities and not bother him about them. No one could object to this if it is clearly understood by all concerned that it is a delegation of authority and *not* usurpation.

Finally some women, just like some men, gain authority by pure subjugation. Figuratively speaking, they beat the poor devil over the head until he gives in and does what they want him to. Besides a headache, which will probably become numb in time, they give him a good start toward an ulcer.

In any event the female influence in business is something to reckon with, whether it comes from a wife, secretary, accountant or woman president. Their health is just as important as the health of the male executive.

HEALTH AND THE WOMAN

For the most part, what has been said here about executive health applies equally and in the same measure to both men and women. She is equally subject to executivitis; has a similar need for a good doctor; is subject to the same tricks of the forebrain (some think more frequently so than the male, but I doubt it); she needs the same sensible balance of work, tension and play; benefits from at least an elementary knowledge of the principles of nutrition and of physiology; is perhaps a little less given to the abuse of tranquilizers and stimulants; and must learn, like all of us, to make the best of what she has.

There are, of course, certain basic and fundamental differences between the male and the female physical machinery and emotional reactions. Chief of these is the procreative apparatus and the differences due to the female vs. the male hormones. This produces differences in body size, contour and physical strength as well as in some psychological reactions. All these differences are obvious. But the over-all differences between the two sexes in terms of function in our present society are nowhere near so great as we used to believe. It is important that society's leaders understand this.

NEW CONCEPT OF WOMEN EXECUTIVES

With the exception of the reigning queens of current history and the "queens" of the arts, sciences and business in our own land, the concept of large numbers of women in high executive positions is relatively new, not older than the last two or three generations. It has come about largely through social and medical advances during that time which have resulted in a new and better status for women. It promises to become more and more common, so let's take a few moments to look at the great changes in women's status in this country over the last seventy-five years, in the hope of foreseeing its future effects.

GRANDMOTHER'S CONTEMPORARIES

Those over fifty have only to remember their grandmothers to recall some of the differences in the role of women then, compared with our daughters today. Few women in the more privileged economic group worked before 1916. Widows and maiden ladies occupied themselves with fancy needlework, music or other forms of art, and a limited but formal type of social activity.

Fainting spells were common and "ladies" were seldom without their smelling salts for use in an emotional situation.

They might be so daring as to play tennis, but always in long white skirts down to the ankles. Horseback riding was acceptable, providing the proper riding habit was worn and they rode side-saddle. Bathing at a public beach was considered daring and called for long black stockings and a bathing suit well fastened around the neck, with skirts to the knees. There was no lolling on the beach. The girls rented a "dressing room" as near the water's edge as possible, and modestly submerged at once. The dash back to the dressing room was especially painful, those clinging bathing suits being so revealing. Skating was respectable but also required skirts down to the ankles.

Yes, that's right boys, no levis for great grandmother, no bikini bathing suits, no skating in tights, and no drum majorettes. There were a few bookkeepers and a few typists, but they were way down the social scale. No women but those from the very poorest classes worked in a factory.

A DIFFERENT SPECIES

The normal physiology of the female was considered a mystery to be shared only among females. Much was made of the menstrual cycle as a cause of disability. For several days a month the young lady was "indisposed" or "not receiving" or "having one of her headaches."

The menopause gave many of them license to be as cantankerous and unreasonable as they pleased for several years. Poor Aunt Mamie was forgiven her foibles because "she's at that age, you know."

Pregnancy was virtually a disgrace. As soon as "it began to show," the woman who should have been a happy potential mother kept out of sight as much as possible and her girl friends referred to her with a significant nod as being in "an interesting condition." Childbirth was indeed a terrifying experience and rightly so, since it carried a death rate nearly ten times that of today.

Sir William Hunter, one of the very first physicians of England to specialize in obstetrics, was the first male ever to deliver a baby for a queen of England. Previously only midwives had been permitted in the bedroom of a queen, or any other woman of England, when she was in labor.

A common cause of real disability in those days, affecting only females, was a peculiar form of anemia called chlorosis. The poor girl was pale as a ghost, fainted more readily than most, and had no energy. She was said to have "gone into a slight decline," and she really was sick.

NEW LIGHT ON A FAMILIAR SPECIES

How different things are for our daughters and granddaughters today. We know now that sunshine and fresh air, together with a well-rounded diet including fresh green vegetables can prevent or cure chlorosis and we almost never see a case any more.

Today, girls faint less frequently than boys, and the bottom has dropped out of the market for smelling salts.

Today, the menstrual cycle is accepted as simple, normal functioning of the female reproductive system, and is seldom the cause of disability. If it is even mildly disabling, the abnormality causing it can be cured nine times out of ten.

Today, pregnancy is looked upon as a joyous occasion, and the way these young mothers jump into their "expecting clothes" during the second month is a delight. They can't wait for it "to show." And the way they meet labor, with chins up, with more and more of them declining anesthesia, so that they may "be there" the moment the baby comes shows how obstetrical techniques have changed. Since the early thirties the birthrate has increased, yet the maternal and infant death death rate has steadily declined. Today, well over ninety per cent of births takes place in well-equipped hospitals and deaths from childbirth are almost as rare as deaths from appendectomies.

Female tennis champions both here and abroad are among the best women athletes the world has produced. Girl swimmers continue to make records in long distance swimming endurance, and fancy skating is as much a woman's sport as a man's. Basketball, soft ball and bowling offer many opportunities for women to excel. A day at the beach for girls and boys alike is really a full day in costumes as near the nude as the law will allow, and with more time spent in resting and sporting on the sand than in the water.

PERHAPS A NEW BREED?

Over one-fourth of those employed in this country today are women, many of them married with children. More and more women are earning prominent places in society as educators, scientists, artists, stateswomen and business executives.

Yes, this is a new breed of women we are seeing today, and I'm all for them. They are far more useful citizens, contributing much more to society than most of their grandmothers and great grandmothers could, and all without smelling salts.

"CHANGE OF LIFE"—MALE AND FEMALE

Discussion of this natural phenomenon was purposely omitted from that portion of the preceeding chapter dealing with diminution of the sexual powers of the male. Not many people realize that males often exhibit some of the same psychological symptoms during this period as do women.

Whereas our grandmothers' contemporaries often made considerable to-do about the "change of life"—in itself a misnomer with sinister overtones—today it is taken in stride by the average healthy woman. Fortunately the woman's menopause is regarded with much less apprehension than it used to be by husband and boss.

I can find no good reason for the formerly common practice in industry of permitting or requiring a woman employee to retire earlier than the men, except that the boss figured he would have had about enough of her menopausal crankiness by the time she was sixty. What a mistake this was.

Women have learned now that they don't have to be miserable or irritable during the gradual cessation of the menses; that "hot flashes" are not serious and can be easily controlled; and even if there has been some little increased nervousness during this time, by the time most of them reach sixty they are really entering the golden age of their lives, more stable and dependable than ever, and usually healthier too.

A "CHANGE," BUT FOR THE BETTER

As with men, women have a strong procreative instinct, whether or not they have ever had a child. As with men, the realization that the reproductive part of their life is about over may be something of a shock, if for no other reason than evidence that they are getting old. This is bound to be a little upsetting to men and women alike. But nowadays we can become adjusted to it more easily than ever before, because of the increased life span and the examples all about us of happy, healthy seventy- and eighty-year-olds.

I once had a patient who went into a real decline on her fortieth birthday. She took to her bed, made her will and prepared to depart this vale of tears. To her, forty years was advanced old age, and she could not expect to live much longer. I told her that I saw no reason for her to die, and that I didn't believe the good Lord would call her until He was ready. After three months, a little disappointed, I thought, she decided maybe the Lord wasn't quite ready for her, so she got out of bed and went on her way rejoicing. She lived to be seventy-eight.

There is good reason for men and women alike feeling a little different when the reproductive years are over. One is psychological, another is due to the need for adjusting to a new balance in the various hormones. The adjustment is made by nature in a relatively short time, but the modern physician can often help nature by supplementing the diminishing hormones for a few months until balance is attained. If this is understood, then there is no need for man or woman to go into a "tizzy" over it. The "tizzy" is more often the cause of discomfort than the changing hormone balance.

WHO'S HEALTHIER?

Who are healthier, men or women? Judging from the death rates, women have it all over men. Their average life-span from birth is almost seven years longer. The latest figures compiled by the Metropolitan Life Insurance Company show the average life span for white women in this country has reached an unprecedented seventy-four years. The average life span from birth for white males in the United States is now a little over sixty-seven. These are provisional figures to be checked later with the U. S. Census Bureau, but they have been remarkably close for many years.

The 1960 death rate for U.S. white males was 10.9 per 100,000; that of females was 8.0. Both death rates have declined markedly in the last fifty years, but women have benefited more than men.

WHAT MORE MEN DIE OF

The causes of death largely responsible for the excess among males are diseases of the heart, blood vessels and kidneys (cardiovascular-renal); cancer, especially of the digestive system, prostate and lung; and accidents, especially at the younger ages, beginning as early as childhood. Women have lower death rates from heart disease and fewer fatal accidents. Women's death rates from cancer of the breast are, of course, higher than men's, but this is largely offset by a marked decrease in deaths from cancer of the uterus and a much lower death rate than men from lung cancer.

A BREAKTHROUGH ON CANCER

This decrease in deaths from cancer of the uterus is one of the truly great breakthroughs in cancer control. It came about through the discovery by Dr. Papanicolaou that smears taken gently from the cervix on a cotton swab, spread on a glass slide and examined under the microscope would sometimes show abnormal cells indicative of early cancer long before the cancer growth had become serious, and while it could still be removed surgically before it spread. There is no question but that this examination, employed at least once a year after age thirty-five, has saved the lives of thousands of women. It would save many thousands more each year if more women could be persuaded to have an annual health check-up which included this simple examination. Many large industries, whose medical department offers and urgently recommends the "Pap Test," find that as many as half of their women employees over thirty-five refuse it.

In one shop with about 1,500 employees, of whom about 400 were women over thirty-five, fewer than 200 would permit the "Pap Test." One of the older women who had consistently refused developed cancer of the cervix and died within the year. She was one of the best liked people in the plant and had many callers during her long hospital stay and lingering illness. She never failed to admonish the girls from the office not only to accept, but to insist on the test when they had their annual examinations. The year following her death over ninety per cent of the women accepted, and they continue to do so ten years later.

So it is with cancer of the breast. As more women learn self-examination of the breasts, either from their physician or by seeing the film on the subject available without charge from the American Cancer Society, more and more are seeking early medical advice for small breast tumors. Most of them are benign. But if they should be found malignant, they can be removed early enough to prevent spread.

Unfortunately, we do not yet know exactly how to use Dr. Papanicolaou's method of examining cells cast off from the body to detect early cancer in the prostate, bladder, lungs, stomach or intestine. He and many others are pursuing studies along this line within the limits of funds available for such research and may soon be able to perfect their intricate techniques. When they do, it is to be hoped that more men as well as women will take advantage of them.

WOMEN TAKE BETTER CARE OF THEMSELVES

There is no question that women live longer than men, and it seems at least partly due to the fact that they take better care of themselves. This has been true only in the last generation. Fifty years ago the excessive hazards of childbirth, cancer and tuberculosis among women caused life insurance companies to limit the number of females they would insure at normal rates.

Unfortunately we do not have figures on the health and longevity of women executives, compared with men executives. We can only make the best of what figures we have on women in general and women in industry.

HOW ABOUT SICK-ABSENCE RATES?

When we look at absence rates due to alleged illness among employed women, compared with men, we might have some doubts as to whether women are healthier. Their sick-absence rates greatly exceed those of men in practically all the studies made to date. This excess of apparent illness holds for all ages of women employees compared with men of similar ages. Some studies show as much as five times more sick-absence among women than among men, with considerable of the excess reported as menstrual disorders.

Over the years our good statisticians have taught me to interpret statistical studies with some discrimination. In examining the figures on female vs. male sick-absence in industry, so many questions come to mind that I am not yet fully convinced women employees are less healthy than men.

ELUSIVE VARIABLES

For one thing, it is tricky business to compare absence rates between industries or sections of the same industry. There are often hidden variables which vitiate the figures. One large industry found the absence rate in its smaller local installations less than half that of their central plant. Everyone was blamed from the Personnel Officer to the supervisorial group to the Medical Division, which was said to be too lenient. The underlying cause was nothing more than a common phenomenon pointed out by the Westinghouse studies many years ago: the more attention employees get from management, the better they work, and coincidentally, the larger the unit under one supervisor, the lower the production and the greater the absence rate.

Another variable which is most elusive is motivation to work. Women wage-earners, not women executives, are often motivated differently from men. Many of them are married, have children and naturally feel that home responsibilities come first. Their earnings are a welcome supplement to the family income but are not so important as taking care of a sick child or preparing a good dinner for the family, or taking advantage of a bargain sale, or even going to the hairdresser. They seem to have many more good reasons than men for not going to work.

The easiest excuse is to allege illness, especially when there is really no good way for even the physician to disprove subjective symptoms. A woman reporting to a male supervisor cannot be too closely questioned concerning the exact nature of her illness, and he cannot be expected to keep tabs on the periodicity of her menstrual cycle. In almost all cases of minor illness causing one to three days' absence, the word of the employee must be taken. Hence, when a child is sick, or the baby sitter is sick, or her hair needs a wash and wave, or she's just tired or has a hangover, it's a simple thing for her not to show up at work, and when questioned on her return to report "bad cold" (no one ever has a simple little cold) or "bad headache" or just "cramps." Whether this is the kind of employee the executive wants is another matter. Sometimes she's the best he can get. She will probably never be a business executive.

These are some of the doubts I have about whether statistics on sick-absence rates among female wage earners in large industries proves that women are less healthy than men. As a longtime health officer of communities as well as industries, I think the only figures you can tie to are the death rates. When a person is dead, there's no question about it. Under civilized conditions in this country, the dead must be decently buried or cremated. Burial or cremation calls for a permit from someone in authority. A permit cannot be obtained until a cause of death is stated.

Again, someone with at least a modicum of judgment must ascribe a cause of death, usually the attending physician or the coroner. The cause of death may not always be fully accurate, but at worst it's an educated guess. It's a lot better than Mary Smith returning to work after two days' absence and answering her supervisor's question with "the cramps," and calling that a statistic.

I recall one overworked, male supervisor years ago who resented the new rule requiring him to report to the personnel division the reason any of his people were absent. Many suspicious ones he was asked to re-question. He finally discovered that one cause of absence was never questioned. So he used it as often as possible on both male and female absentees. It was dysmenorrhea.

My own feeling, therefore, is that women of today are really healthier than men. In this country we find them generally acceptable for almost any kind of employment except heavy labor. In the communes and armies of the socialist republics, even this distinction is wiped out.

WHO IS MORE EMOTIONAL?

Are women more affected by their emotions than men? Well, here, I can't prove that they are not. In fact, I share the general impression of many others that they are. But even if this be true, is it a cause of condemnation in business? In extreme cases, of course, a highly emotional woman executive could be a disaster in a big office. But so are highly emotional men, of whom there are many. The fact is that highly emotional people, usually meaning those who have not learned to direct their emotions into constructive channels, are not usually attracted to positions of high executive authority anyway. If they are, either by circumstances or misjudgment, the give-and-take—often the rough-and-tumble—of business life usually drives them out.

I can suggest merely that executives who must decide between a man or a woman for an executive position apply the same criteria to each. One essential requirement for anyone with executive responsibilities is the maturity that comes with emotional stability.

Some men find it distasteful to be subordinate to a woman in a business or profession. There are occasions in which this may be justified. I submit, however, that much of this is prejudice. One has only to look at the outstanding success of many of our women college presidents, the smooth functioning of many elementary and secondary schools with women principals, the remarkable ability of many women superintendents in hospitals and the usually efficient functioning of many businesses with women presidents to realize that not all women are over-emotional.

To summarize, we have in this country during the last two generations begun to produce a new type of woman—one who has cast aside her Victorian restrictions and the confines of a separate world for females. She has demonstrated ample capacity for education, political leadership, good judgment, and especially superior concern with human welfare. She has shown that her health, both mental and physical, is as good as that of men, or even better, thanks both to medical and sociological advances. She proves to have important values to society even beyond those of child-bearing, child-rearing and husband nurture. She is no longer man's chattel, but rather his valued assistant and partner—one whose capacity for love of humanity often exceeds his; one who will often help soften his harsher decisions; and one whose new participation in local and world affairs may help turn the male's tragic traditions of war and destruction toward a more peaceful world.

CHAPTER

10

EMPLOYEES' HEALTH

ARE YOU AN "ULCER MAKER"?

I HOPE that by now I have made it sufficiently clear that the health of executives, both male and female, deserves attention. Much depends on their good health—not only their own success, but the success of their business, whatever it may be. Upon the success of the business depends, oftentimes, the security, safety, well-being and good health of many employees. It is appallingly true that maladministration and bad interpersonal relations on the part of the boss can cause illness among some of his subordinates. There certainly are "ulcer makers" among some of our executives, and no one knows how many accidents and other disabilities are basically caused by bad handling of the employee by his superiors. Such bad handling is more likely to occur when the boss himself is not in good health. For this reason alone, as well as many others, his health deserves the best attention he can learn to give it.

NATURE HELPS THOSE WHO HELP THEMSELVES

Maintaining and improving health depends primarily on the personal initiative of the individual. Nothing else, except perhaps Mother Nature's chance arrangement of the molecules in his genes, can create good health for him. With this one exception, it cannot be forced upon him. It cannot be purchased in pill or bottle. It is attained only by acquiring health intelligence, following sensible living habits such as I have tried to outline, and taking advantage of the best medical advice. This much is essential.

Reflecting on the fact that his own poor health may endanger the health and safety of his subordinates is rather a chilling thought for the executive. But his poor health may be reflected in poor personnel policies, and other bad handling of employees. This in turn can cause fright, anger, frustration or vindictiveness. As we have seen with the executive himself, when these emotions are too intense or prolonged, they can lead to that old conflict between the primitive instinct toward fight-or-flight, and the more intelligent desire to preserve the peace and retain a much-needed job. This conflict is a direct pathway to illness and accident.

MISMANAGEMENT MEANS MISHANDLING EMPLOYEES

There are other ways of mishandling employees with even more direct consequences. These may be caused more by the executive's ignorance than his poor health. It is now pretty well established by law, embellished by the Workmen's Compensation Boards and Commissions in this country, that the employer is responsible for providing a work-place that is safe and healthy. He is severely penalized in his compensation insurance rates if a workman is injured or made ill, not only as a result of, but "in the course of" his employment. Within the last year, rulings have also included mental illness developed "in the course of" employment. Later in this chapter we shall see some of the disasters which resulted from disregard of these tenets, especially in smaller businesses.

If the executive will reflect a little beyond his proper concern for his own health and his legal obligations to employees, he may agree that good health has become almost a right in this country and that no one should be denied it for lack of knowledge or lack of means to obtain it, or by being assigned a job that harms him. Some employers, especially in small businesses, are unwilling to concern themselves with these obligations. Others, under the pressures of the bargaining table, have been forced to assume some responsibility for health safeguards as well as medical care. There can be no question about the recent trends toward employee health and safety in these labor sessions.

WILL THE JOB DESTROY THE WORKMAN?

What this all leads up to is that today's industry has come a long way from the common disregard for employees' health and safety prior to the industrial revolution of one hundred years ago. In this country, today, all employers have legal obligations to safeguard their employees' health and safety, and most employers voluntarily assume humanitarian and moral obligations as well.

They are beginning to see that costs of industrial health programs are negligible compared with the resulting reduced absenteeism, lowered compensation costs and improved morale.

The lack of knowledge concerning the health and safety of workers prior to the mid-Nineteenth century is hard for us to comprehend today. Bernardino Ramazzini (1633-1714) is generally regarded as the first physician to study the effects of occupation on health. He visited many workmen at their places of work; gravediggers, sewer inspectors, potters, glass-blowers and mirror-makers all came under his scrutiny. Nearly all mirror-makers of Florence eventually succumbed to mercury poisoning, and one shudders at Ramazzini's vivid description of their physical suffering, mental deterioration and early death. Looking at their disfigured faces in their own beautiful handiwork, he says they cursed themselves and the day they were born. It's hard to realize that they had no other choice but to follow their trade to make a living. The average life-span of workmen in these days was probably less than thirty years.

THE SOLUTION IN LARGE INDUSTRY

The experience of many large industries, some as far back as fifty years ago, has shown beyond question that an in-plant industrial health program is a necessity. Let us see briefly what it is, its results, and how its benefits may be obtained for small as well as large businesses.

The Council on Occupational Health of the American Medical Association, 535 North Dearborn Street, Chicago 10, Illinois, has described the "meeds and bounds" of an industrial health program, as approved by its Board of Trustees and House of Delegates. This is available in pamphlet form at no cost, and is familiar to most state and county medical societies. Briefly it recommends:

Establishing an industrial health conservation program which concentrates on preventive rather than curative services. If there is another program to provide medical and hospital care for sick employees and their dependents, it should be administered separately under a separate account. The medical director may be placed in charge of both, but if so, he "wears two hats" and operates each program on a different budget.

PROPER PURPOSES

The purposes of the health conservation program are to:

(a) assist the employer with the proper selection and placement of a new employee in a job which will not impair his health or endanger others;

(b) to make regular inspections of the entire plant to discover and help management eliminate or minimize hazards to safety either in equipment or practices, and hazards to health through unnecessary exposure to toxic substances or extremes of temperature, barometric pressure, light, vibration or noise, and to assure proper sanitation in water, food and milk supplied by the employer, with proper disposal of sewage and industrial wastes;

(c) to be familiar with the real and potential harmfulness of all materials used and by-products formed and their proper handling;

(d) to safeguard the health of all employees through periodic health examinations and adequate counseling following the examination, and at any other time the employee has health problems;

(e) to refer employees with definite or suspected illness to a physician of their choice for their treatment, helping the employee obtain an appointment and cooperating with such physician during the employee's disability;

(f) to render first-aid to all injured, including minor injuries;

(g) to give prompt care within the limits desired by the employer to all workmen's compensation cases, i.e., those injured during and in the course of employment;
(h) to establish friendly relationships with practicing physicians and with health and welfare agencies in the community from whom employees may need assistance;
(i) to organize and conduct a program of health and safety education among employees and their families.

MEANS OF ACCOMPLISHMENT

The means of accomplishing such a program are first to obtain a qualified medical director, preferably one who specializes in occupational medicine and is so certified by the American Board of Preventive Medicine. If no such specialist is available, or the industry is too small to justify a full-time physician, then seek one who takes a special interest in industrial medicine and is willing to devote a specified amount of time to work in the plant. The local medical society can often be helpful in finding the right man. Experience shows that the physician who is merely "on call" or who sees only the employees in his office is not usually satisfactory. The full-time medical director in the larger plants may need one or more full-time or part-time physician assistants.

Many small businesses start their program by hiring a nurse. She should have special training or experience in industrial health work, as recommended in the pamphlets prepared by the American Association of Industrial Nurses, 170 East 61 Street, New York 21, N.Y., and the Industrial Nursing Section of the American Nurses Association, 2 Park Avenue, New York 16, N.Y. Too often she is selected for her good looks or because she did satisfactory private duty nursing in the boss's family. A good industrial nurse working alone, with only a doctor on call will be very valuable. But what she can do is limited by law in the medical and the nursing practice acts of each state. The employer who expects her to exceed these limitations puts himself and the nurse in legal jeopardy. It is much better to have at least a part-time medical director who spends regular hours in the plant dispensary and who gives her standing orders, taking legal responsibility for the over-all program.

Other small plants may start with a part-time first-aid man, preferably one who has an up-to-date certificate from the American Red Cross first-aid course and who is familiar with safety programs. He, too, can be very valuable—in fact, almost essential—but his value is greatly enhanced when he becomes a member of the "industrial health team" working with the doctor and nurse and such other team-members as are needed.

THE INDUSTRIAL HEALTH TEAM

The medical director chosen should select the nurse who will be his invaluable assistant. Besides the nurse and safety man, he may have need of other members for his health team, depending upon the hazards of the industry. Among the first of these may be an industrial hygienist, either full- or part-time. Industrial hygienists are people specially trained in chemistry or physics or industrial toxicology or sanitary, acoustical, ventilation, illumination or nuclear engineering. The doctor, nurse or safety man may locate a hazard, injuries from which involve management liability, but an expert in industrial hygiene may be needed to design and supervise corrective measures. These may include hoods and exhaust vents for control of harmful dusts or noxious gases, protection from radiation hazards, sequestration and insulation for excessively noisy operations, etc.

I recall one large airplane service hangar which was among the first to be equipped with an X-ray machine to detect flaws from metal fatigue. Although instructed by the dealer on its safe installation and use, the operators were changed several times and grew careless. Then an efficiency expert, knowing nothing of the necessary precautions, speeded up inspections by moving the machine from place to place. This resulted in X-rays being bounced around the entire hangar exposing all the workers to excessive and dangerous dosage. With the backing of top management, an industrial hygienist, expert in nuclear physics, designed a fool-proof shield for the machine. We could only hope it had been done in time to forestall a score of compensation claims for X-ray injury.

A PLACE TO WORK

In addition to appropriate personnel, according to the American Medical Association brochure, the medical director will need a dispensary of some sort in which he and the nurse may work, and which becomes the company's "health center." It should be centrally located, well lighted and ventilated, with moisure-proof floors and walls easy to clean, and should provide privacy. Its equipment need not be luxurious but must provide the doctor and nurse with the tools of their profession.

CONFIDENTIAL NATURE OF MEDICAL RECORDS

Medical records, according to the American Medical Association and all the ethical principles of the medical profession, must be strictly confidential between the medical department and the individual employee. They are kept under lock and key and may not be divulged by anyone connected with the medical department except with the consent of the patient. Management is entitled to know who is disabled, how serious the disability is, and its probable duration, but not necessarily the diagnosis except with the consent of the disabled. Management is also entitled to know when one of their key men is stricken with a serious or progressively disabling illness. This is practically always worked out by the experienced and tactful physician who has little difficulty in eventually persuading the patient to give his consent, or to report it himself. Some illnesses and much that goes on between the physician and his patient is privileged information, and divulgence of it could damage the patient. Indeed, if this were not the case, few employees would avail themselves of the medical department's services since, theoretically at least, none of them want their personal health problems to become generally known throughout the plant.

While it is important for management to understand the reasons for confidentiality of industrial medical records, this is rarely a troublesome problem. Nine times out of ten the patient himself tells people or readily gives the doctor permission to do so. Nevertheless, there are occasions, such as pregnancy in an unmarried woman, or venereal disease, when the physician must protect the best interests of the patient while at the same time protecting other employees and the employer. This is one reason why not all physicians are entirely satisfactory in industry.

CO-OPERATION OF LOCAL DOCTORS

It is important for the industrial physician to be on good terms with fellow-physicians in the community. This is difficult if he is looked upon as an unfair competitor who treats the patients of the other doctors free, being paid to do so by the industry. If, however, he can honestly say that he is employed to safeguard the health of their patients who happen to work in the industry, and that he is there primarily to assure a safe and healthful working environment and to help keep employees on the job, that when he finds any of them ill they are not treated by him but promptly referred to their own doctor and that he will be glad to cooperate with their own physician by furnishing the employee's work history and any physical findings or laboratory tests he has, then the private physician finds he has nothing to complain about and becomes co-operative.

His co-operation is often a great help in persuading his patient not to abuse sick benefits or to prolong his disability unnecessarily. This is the reason the American Medical Association urges limiting the actual treatment given by the industrial physician to emergency first aid, and minor ailments for which the employee would not ordinarily consult his physician. Most sick benefit plans permit free choice of physician with some exceptions where the large industry provides complete hospital and medical care through company physicians and company hospitals. Thus, even though the company physician may be responsible for administering the sick benefit plan, he may still expect the full co-operation of his local colleagues because he is still not in competition with them. It is well recognized by the Blue Cross-Blue Shield groups as well as the private health insurance companies that the attitude of the local medical profession can make or break any health insurance plan. If the doctors are willing so to demean themselves as to enter into a conspiracy with their patient to get all they possibly can from the "Blues" or the insurance companies, then no insurance plan can long remain solvent.

I have had many occasions to be proud of the medical profession when doctor-patient conspiracy has threatened an otherwise sound health insurance plan in a given locality and the county medical society has come to the rescue. The approach by the insurance company and the remedy by the local medical society fall into pretty much the same pattern:

The insurance company prepares exact figures showing how much greater the claim-rate is in that locality compared with similar insured groups in other localities, and with nationwide averages. They then invite the members of the local medical society, or if that is too large, the officers of the society and the nearby doctors who have been signing most of the claim papers, to a good evening dinner in a pleasant club or restaurant. After the dinner we say that we of the insurance company have come to learn from them and to seek their advice on a troublesome problem which is having adverse effects on their patients, the major employers and perhaps on themselves. The figures are then presented clearly and dispassionately. The possible necessity of withdrawing or curtailing benefits, or of the industry being obliged to transfer its operations to another community are pointed out. We conclude by saying something to the effect that it's a serious problem for all of us, but mainly for the local doctors. "What do you advise?"

Then comes the hardest part, which is to say no more. The dead silence often seems endless. The "hot heads" are usually the first to speak. They may damn the insurance company, or the employer or the low characters chosen to work for the company. Not infrequently they get to damning each other. There may be an hour or more of "free-for-all."

Eventually the cooler-headed leaders, of whom there is always a surprising number, begin to take over. They calm the troubled waters, humorously but effectively chide themselves and the others for letting things come to such a state of affairs and begin to present constructive suggestions. Ultimately they form a committee to which the insurer, the employer or the individual patient may refer disputed or questionable cases. This is just what we were all hoping for. It is their remedy, not ours. Following this action we have seen claim rates decrease as much as fifty per cent.

A FRILL OR A NECESSITY?

All this may sound like a big order to the executive whose business has not had a medical department, or who thought his business was too small for such frills.

I have seen so many health and financial disasters resulting from lack of medical service, in businesses both large and small, that it is my conviction no business or industry regardless of size can afford to be without competent medical counsel. The cost of a well-run industrial health program, excluding the cost of any sick-benefit plan which is really in lieu of wages, is not prohibitive. It ranges from $25 to $200 per employee per year, depending on how elaborate it is, how frequent and how serious the operational hazards may be, and how the books are kept. It is a proper charge against the costs of doing business since it protects and enhances the health of employees, often reduces absenteeism and workmen's compensation costs, and is an important aid to morale.

DISASTER, BOTH HEALTH AND FINANCIAL

Granted that the problem is a little more difficult in the smaller businesses, several satisfactory methods are now available and they will be discussed in a moment.

But first let me give just a few typical examples, taken from my own experiences, of health and financial disaster occurring in industry because of lack of medical advice.

A large terminal on a seaway employing an average of 500, sometimes had 1,000 workers, sometimes only fifty. There was a cross-connection between the drinking water supply and the fire-fighting water supply which was pumped directly from the river below in emergency. Such cross-connections are now illegal in most states, but management was either unaware of this or chose to ignore it. Through some accident of ignorance or carelessness an employee opened the cross-connecting valve, which remained open for three days when nearly a thousand men were working on the docks. The drinking water supply was thus flooded with river water which was heavily polluted with untreated sewage.

Employees complained that the drinking water was cloudy and tasted slightly salty especially at high tide, the terminal being just slightly above tide-water. Nothing was done about it, however, until the third day when about 300 employees failed to show up for work because of dysentery. Several hundred more complained of diarrhea but came to work. The dysentery cases were reported to the health department as required by law. The health officer and his sanitary engineer located the open cross-connection at once, closed the valve and flushed out the pipes. Two to three weeks later cases of typhoid fever began to appear. Altogether there were thirty-six cases of typhoid and four deaths among the thousand employees. (This was before we had antibiotics for treatment.) All disabilities due to dysentery and typhoid and the four deaths were held to be compensable. The cost of paying these claims nearly threw the employer into bankruptcy. Any physician, nurse or even a safety man would have investigated the turbid drinking water at once, thus saving a great many victims.

Some years ago I was inspecting the largest industry in a small city, employing about 800 persons. They had no medical director, nurse or safety man. The business had grown rapidly and the plant "housekeeping" was terrible. Poor housekeeping is usually associated with a high accident rate, which they were having. That's why I was sent there by their insurer. The stairs were cluttered with cans, boxes and tools; the floors were dirty and slippery in spots where fluids had been spilled and not wiped up. Windows were dirty and lighting often inadequate. A strong odor of some solvent pervaded the entire plant. In one department using this solvent about half the employees complained of dermatitis on their hands.

To my horror I found a large open barrel of the solvent at the foot of a stairway. "No smoking" signs were posted all about and the rule was enforced on this floor, but not elsewhere in the building. I urged the superintendent to move and cover this barrel at once, then submitted a number of other recommendations including the employment of a part-time physician and a full-time industrial nurse.

En route home the next day I read in the papers that the entire plant had burned to the ground, killing two and injuring twenty. The vat of solvent had exploded when one of the men, preparing to observe the no smoking rule, tapped out his pipe on the stair-rail directly above the open barrel.

Their credit was good enough to permit them to rebuild a modern factory and eventually regain their customers, but nothing could restore the lives lost or the time lost by the injured. A modicum of safety-consciousness and common sense, even without a doctor or nurse, would have prevented this tragedy.

During the lay-off while the factory was rebuilding, the forty or more with dermatitis filed compensation claims and got awards. When the new factory opened, a competent part-time physician and a full-time nurse was hired. With a simple prescription for a protective cream and instruction and supervision on its proper use from the nurse, the dermatitis was stopped. The solvent was changed to something less dangerous and irritating and it was used in a closed vat under an exhaust hood.

Dust and air in certain proportions are spontaneously combustible. Operators of grain elevators and flour mills are well aware of this. But at least one manufacturer of plastic dice and dominoes was not. He employed twenty-four girls and two men in a second floor single large room to shape and spot the rectangles and cubes. Shaping involved a row of grinding wheels against which a jig pressed and turned the product. No suction ventilation was provided and the dust cloud filled the room, especially in winter with the windows closed. The proprietor had been assured by the supplier of the plastic that this dust was no more harmful than sawdust, which may have been true. But he knew nothing about the combustibility of this or any other dust.

One winter afternoon the whole room blew up. Three persons

were killed outright, three died later of extensive burns, and not one of the twenty-seven people in the room escaped burns. The proprietor was bankrupt and went out of business. Having fewer than twenty-five women employees, his small new factory had not yet been inspected by the State Department of Labor. He admitted that the girls often complained about the dust, but he reassured them with the word of the supplier of the raw material.

A retail butcher thought he saw an opportunity to "clean up" on the holiday trade when he found a turkey grower who was selling off his entire flock at half price, saying he was going out of business. The butcher bought well over a thousand birds and hired ten poultry butchers to dress them. All went well, seemingly, and he "cleaned up"—almost.

Within the month six of the ten butchers took sick and one finally died. They all had ornithosis, formerly known as "parrot fever." It is a virus-like disease common to many species of birds besides parrots, especially parakeets, canaries and turkeys. It is easily transmitted to humans by inhaling the dust from the dried feces or through small cuts in the hands while eviscerating poultry. So far as we know, it is not transmitted to man through eating the cooked meat.

What this medically ignorant or medically oblivious little butcher didn't know, or chose to ignore, was that he had purchased the remnants of a flock which had suffered a severe epidemic of ornithosis. Those birds remaining alive were saved by feeding an antibiotic, but many of them still carried the live causative agent in their lungs, livers, and digestive tracts; hence, they were still infectious. He claimed he didn't know either, that this same "bargain" had been declined by the Army Quartermaster responsible for supplying the regional military posts. The Quartermaster *did* have the benefit of advice from the medical corps. By the time the butcher had paid the disability and death claims assessed against him, he went out of business too. Today, thank goodness, that State has a modern poultry inspection law.

Apart from these individual cases, there are many over-all health problems which periodically engulf industry as a whole, or groups of related industries. They arise from new products or by-products, or from the development of new methods, the effects of which on human beings may remain unknown for a time. But if they prove harmful they hit like an avalanche and everyone seems in trouble. We know a lot today about preventing or ameliorating the harmful effects of lead, mercury, phosphorus, radiation, inhalation of finely divided silica dust and many other common industrial hazards.

It seems only yesterday, however, when the Public Health Service and the Bureau of Mines completed their studies on dust inhalation and proved beyond a doubt that the slowly progressive, eventually disabling and often fatal "miner's lung," or silicosis, is caused by long exposure to dust containing high percentages of very fine particles of silica dioxide. It often led to, or was accompanied by tuberculosis, or enormous enlargement of the heart, or both. For many years it was the cause of prolonged disability and early death among hard rock miners, "sand hogs" and stone cutters. They were not unlike, though not quite as bad off as Ramazzini's mirror-makers—no one knew why so many sickened and died.

Once silicosis proved to be of occupational origin, mine operators, tunnel contractors, suppliers of carved stone, were all in trouble. Compensation cases flooded employers at the same time they had to install expensive apparatus for dust control. Many individual operators went under but eventually the afflicted industry recovered and many lives were saved.

A similar but smaller disastrous avalanche occurred with the more recent mining and fabrication of beryllium. Before we knew it, men exposed to certain forms of beryllium sickened and died with some mysterious lung disease. The doctors and industrial hygienists were on the job a little quicker this time and control measures were soon adopted. But many compensation claims are still being paid those totally disabled with berylliosis.

Among the new potential avalanches which hang over the heads of industry today are uranium injury, chromium poisoning and occupational deafness.

Some uranium miners are developing some queer disabilities which may be related to the peculiar effects of exposure to the raw ore, or carelessness in handling the refined product.

We have long known that peculiar, punched-out ulcers of the

skin, difficult to heal, occur among chrome workers. We have learned to control most of them by protective devices and special definitive treatment. It begins to appear, however, that chromium miners and others occupationally exposed have a higher rate of lung cancer than the general population. It is not yet certain that this is a cause and effect relationship, but if it should be, which way do we turn for preventive measures?

The occupational deafness avalanche has already struck in many compensation jurisdictions. It may be worse than silicosis before we're through.

Only a few years ago it was discovered that continuous exposure to excessive noise causes permanent impairments of hearing. There can be no doubt of this. But how to distinguish between this kind of deafness and that which often occurs naturally as we get older is a problem. Meanwhile many compensation boards are granting awards for any kind of deafness. This was discussed in Chapter Six but is brought up here again as another example of how the employer may be adding to his compensation costs by unwittingly injuring a workman's hearing. He will avoid this if he obtains and heeds advice from a good industrial physician or industrial hygienist. Occupational deafness *can* be prevented.

I could cite many other examples illustrating the importance of medical counsel to every employer, large or small. Few businesses today of any size are operated without advice from attorneys, engineers, architects and accountants. Over 90 per cent of the employees in this country work for companies with less than 500 on the payroll. I doubt if 10 per cent of such employers realize their need for medical counsel. True, competent, part-time medical service has been hard to obtain in the past. But there are a number of good ways to do it now.

GOOD HEALTH SERVICE FOR SMALL INDUSTRY

In some cities a group of highly competent specialists in occupational health have banded together to provide first class service to the smaller firms in their area. Charges are made on the basis of number of employees and services given. Industries with few hazards may require the physician to visit the plant only one half day a week, and the nurse two days a week. An expert industrial hygienist may be called in when needed to deal with special problems. Meanwhile the physician is always on call for emergencies.

In a half day a week at the plant, the physician can, with the help of a nurse and a clerk, do pre-employment examinations and periodic health examinations for the older employees (including the executives) to the extent of about twenty-five a month and still have time to inspect the plant periodically and set aside time at each visit to counsel employees having health problems. This is an excellent arrangement for the smaller businesses. It should be more commonly available in more cities. Competent industrial physicians would be more encouraged to organize such services if a group of small industries agreed to support it. Physicians are reticent about soliciting business, but are glad to respond when called.

THE PART-TIME INDUSTRIAL PHYSICIAN

Another way for small industries to provide themselves with a satisfactory health program is to obtain the part-time services of a physician who is not necessarily a specialist in occupational medicine, but who is interested in it, and willing to devote part of his time to this type of practice. These men are usually general practitioners or internists, occasionally surgeons. With some study of the medical literature on industrial hygiene and especially if the industry will make it possible for him to attend one or two meetings of industrial physicians each year, he can do a satisfactory and creditable job.

Like any other good general practitioner, he can take care of all the usual medical problems, resorting to consultation with a specialist when unusual problems arise. Again, an industrial nurse, either full-time or part-time will greatly enhance the value of the physician's services, and the nurse's services will be greatly enhanced by some clerical help.

Most local or state medical societies keep a roster of their members who are interested and qualified in industrial medicine and are glad to help the employer find a satisfactory physician.

Two things should be clearly understood. The first is that the physician will regularly spend a certain amount of time in the plant where he can become familiar with the personnel and with the materials and processes used, can give personal attention to the work of the nurse, first-aid and safety men; that he will do the physical examinations in the plant rather than at his office, and that he will be on-call for emergencies.

The second is that he will neither solicit nor accept as a private patient any employee of the plant. This may seem harsh, and is sometimes hard to abide by, but if it is not done it puts him in unfair competition with his fellow-physicians, to which they have a right to object. This kind of competition will alienate the good will of the local physicians, which is often important, since they largely determine the duration of disability of the employees who may be their patients.

THE "ON-CALL" PHYSICIAN

The least satisfactory way to provide the small industry with a physician's services, but still better than nothing, is to designate a physician who will be on-call in case of emergency and who will do pre-employment and periodic health examinations only in his office. This gives him no opportunity to become familiar with plant personnel, materials or processes. It means he is examining applicants for jobs he knows little about, and is checking up on the health of employees whose job hazards and stresses he cannot assess. He often tends to leave too much responsibility to the nurse which subjects her and the employer to liability for mistakes in the treatment and handling of emergencies. Still, this arrangement is better than nothing.

THE PART-TIME INDUSTRIAL NURSE

If the employed group is very small and the employer disposed to provide nothing more than a little part-time nursing service, arrangements may often be made with the local Visiting Nurse Association to send in a specially qualified nurse for an hour or so, two or three times a week. Her charges will be on an hourly basis and are just enough to cover the cost, the V.N.S. being a non-profit organization. She will be helpful to employees with health problems in seeing that they are referred to the proper place, will render first aid and will, if requested, call on employees who are disabled at home to see that they are receiving proper care. Such solicitude by the employer is often a morale-builder.

Such a nurse—in fact, any nurse—should not be used as a truant officer to spy on the absentee with alleged disability by calling at his home. This is a waste of nurse-power which is, and will be for some time to come, in extremely short supply in this country. If the employer feels that he must have a truant officer, it should not be a nurse.

Finally, there are at least three ways the small industry can obtain competent medical advice on special problems without making permanent additions to the payroll.

PRIVATE CONSULTANTS

One is to engage the temporary services of a private consultant, of whom there are now a goodly number over the country. Their names and special skills may usually be obtained from the state or county medical society or by writing the nearest medical school, or the Industrial Medical Association 28 East Jackson Boulevard, Chicago 4, Illinois, or the Council on Occupational Medicine of the American Medical Association, 535 North Dearborn Street, Chicago 10, Illinois. They are comparatively high priced but are worth it. When one needs a specialist in any professional field, the best is none too good.

AID FROM HEALTH DEPARTMENTS

Another way to get sound advice on an industrial health problem in some states and cities is to request help from the local or state health department. Not all health departments have an industrial health division, but when they do they are usually very good. A preliminary survey and advisory service is usually rendered without cost and it is done skillfully and discretely. With the exception of New York State and Massachusetts in which the excellent industrial health bureau is part of the Department of Labor, other health departments are not usually directly concerned with enforcement of labor laws dealing with working conditions.

When the problem is serious and especially if it is highly complicated and affects a whole industry scattered in several states, the state health department has access to the Public Health Service Division of Occupational Health where the very best industrial physicians, engineers, hygienists and nurses are available.

THE INSURANCE CARRIER

A third way to get sound advice on health problems, and perhaps this should be the first to be considered, is to request advice from the company which carries the firm's group health, or workmen's compensation insurance. Many of these companies, though not all, have very competent health and safety experts on their staff and are prepared to render advisory service at little or no cost in order to help the employer reduce claim-rates.

L'ENVOI

In final review, I am at peace with what has been written here. It is my best effort on this subject as of this date. Tomorrow my mind may change on some subjects, for who can foresee the new discoveries just over the horizon in this rapidly changing world of the most scientific medicine we have ever known? But today, it is the best advice I can offer, based on my own years of practice, study and observation.

Perhaps I should warn the reader that some of my professional colleagues will be critical of various opinions expressed here, and for rather interesting reasons. For fifty centuries the practice of medicine was a strange combination of empirical observation, superstition and religion. The physician's final opinion had to be based upon his own personal experiences. Since no two medical experiences are ever exactly alike, opinions differed more often than they agreed. In fact, what to do when doctors disagree is still a vexatious question for many a patient with an obscure illness.

More exact science has developed in medicine during the last century than in all the other forty nine put together. But there is still much about the healthy and the ailing human body that is unknown—so much in fact, that there is plenty of room for many honest differences of opinion amongst good physicians.

To those physicians whose opinions on a given subject may differ from mine, my highest respect. I am sure they will find other opinions which coincide with theirs. But it is my fond hope that they may forego the usual sport of some physicians, who condemn in toto, when really disagreeing only on one or two points, and these often minor.

As a closing reprise, let me just remind you to be of good cheer. The human body is a wondrous mechanism, tending invariably, and with amazing persistence, to right itself when thrown off balance. Living cells, injured by trauma or disease, will heal themselves or be replaced by new tissue if at all possible, so that the total mechanism will continue to function in some fashion. Even the disordered mind, when there is no actual damage to the brain cells, will tend to right itself again when given half a chance.

This inherent healing power of living tissue was never better epitomized than by Ambroise Paré, the wise and observing 16th Century surgeon to the armies of four French kings. "I dressed him, but God healed him," he is reported to have said of the soldiers whose wounds he treated successfully.

In the average doctor's practice today, the majority of his sick patients recover. He assures or hastens recovery in far more cases than Ambroise Paré could because science has given him such a vast array of specific cures and effective treatments. He, too, has learned that in most cases, nature is working on his side. He has learned, and will teach his patient, how to take advantage of nature's self-healing tendencies.

To maintain and enhance our good health, we have only two major obligations. One is to understand the basic principles of what we are made of, and how we function. The other is to learn to adapt ourselves to our own unique and individual environment, or to escape it in ways that will not injure our structure and functioning. The environment to which each of us must adjust is not merely weather and geography. It is mainly other people. Successful adjustment in our relationships with others will usually spare us the disabling "tricks of the forebrain."

If this book makes these obligations a little easier for the leaders of our society—our men and women executives—it will have served its purpose.

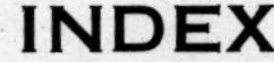

INDEX

INDEX